KUNDALINI AWAKENING
FOR BEGINNERS

Activate Your Kundalini Energy and Increase Your Psychic Abilities
with Yoga Breathing Exercises and Chakra Meditation Poses
to Strengthen Your Body, Mind, and Soul

Willow Kumar

TABLE OF CONTENTS

INTRODUCTION

Kundalini is a term that is spreading like wildfire throughout spiritual cycles. People just accept it as a fact without questioning what it means in any meaningful way. Hence, in this book we'll explore the meaning of "Kundalini."

Kundalini can only be understood by first imagining God or the origin of the cosmos. You must be able to visualize the cosmos as a collection of continents and comprehend the entire universe as a united section and limitless ocean. Like a zygote or a fungus, the cosmos is incredibly scattered in this way. This contributes to the emergence of polarity in the cosmos. Men and women, conscious and unconscious, life and death, remain in opposition, and this polarity must be maintained. The dichotomy of death and life gives birth to the emergence of Kundalini since Kundalini means "life force energy." Kundalini is the polar opposite of death, an empty, lifeless body. As a result, it is critical to comprehend this.

The term "death" may signify various things to the human race. The physical death that humans experience is only a shift in perspective; it is not death in how we think of it. Kundalini is merely the universe's animating defect. It is the inverse of the prefix of every biological form, regardless of dimension. It may be found in beans as well as devils and spirits. Life now shares many traits with death. Simply said, one of the qualities of Kundalini is animation. Animations include both stillness and movement.

As a result, Kundalini can be either static or moving. In other words, anything that has been stiffed might yet be alive. Kundalini's attributes include growth, change, response, reproduction, and creativity. Most of the difficulties we face in the universe are caused by the fact that polarity exists inside us; we do not have integration between life and death.

So, see yourself as a part of this united awareness, implying that you are a fragment of life's polarity. Another way to think about Kundalini is to visualize a limitless ocean. You are inextricably linked to God or the cosmos. Your existence and body are made up of the same energy as God, which presents itself in the physical form of life force energy.

When someone imagines themselves, they envision a life force energy known as the soul. Others envision the soul like a cup of energy, just as they perceive the body as a column of energy. They see a stream of energy that simply creates and expresses physicality in actuality.

One of the soul's characteristics is to transcend life and death. For example, vision must alter before death; else, you would be unable to comprehend death. This signifies that life is just one facet of the soul, and you should realize that you can't have both the soul and life simultaneously. You can die because you are the source of life, implying you are a Kundalini.

To mention energy levels just above physicality, the life force stream of energy materializes in the physical body, allowing a man who was in the physical body to organize himself into radiance and chakras, which are the fundamental structure and energy blueprint of the physical body. To clearly understand this, consider the ancient Hindu sages.

The Hindus refer to the energy centers as chakras since each chakra is assigned to a specific place of the human body. It was formerly thought that humans could feed life force energy into the various sections of the body via the chakras. The chakras were viewed as having the ability to accept and emit energy in multiple ways.

Now, Kundalini is merely a Hindi term that comes from the spiritual world of yoga and may be translated as "the coiled one." The Ancient World believed that the energy might be latent, and if it was inactive and lying towards the base of the spine or the backside of the root chakra, it meant that the chakra was out of alignment.

It's easy to imagine the latent energy these people will absorb as coiled-up snakes at the base of the spine based on how the energy feels in the body as it moves.

Detecting Kundalini in parts of the body associated with chakra is much easier because those parts of the body are associated with physicality and sensation. It will also start moving if you allow your Kundalini energy and the flow of life force energy to animate your body to move like a stream, resembling a snake.

Energy rushes through when the Kundalini can operate at a lower energy level. The radiance and physical strength will be adequate, with the spine running as one current, to connect the lower and top chakras. If you master your Kundalini energy, you will be able to purposefully enable gushes of life force energy to flow through your body. It also has a property that is quite comparable to liquid fire.

One of the most important arguments against Kundalini is that it is nothing more than dormant energy. Kundalini does not disappear when you die. Instead, it remains static. Kundalini is not dormant energy that must be awoken; rather, it is always awake and functioning. Energy may be turned down. Kundalini encounters suppression as a form of resistance. When Kundalini provides space for other types of awareness that are banned or halted by observing objects, it tends to be still.

Kundalini will be quiet when consciousness has to be in a condition of observation. Kundalini must become still when fought with free will since that is where it derives its consciousness. If someone is in the process of determining whether or not they wish to be physically alive, their Kundalini will be still. For example, if a person is in a coma, Kundalini will stay motionless.

The sensation of Kundalini, which drives it into a state of stillness through genuine existence, will be unpleasant. The first question you should ask yourself when you start feeling this way is whether or not you are fighting life. The opposition is simply known as resistance. You could think of it as any opposing force you are familiar with. You must recognize that there is a reason your body is expressing itself in this way.

Kundalini includes a man's creative potential, so you should be concerned about how you are denying your authenticity and purpose for being here. Yoga breathing exercises, self-surrender, and meditation, along with all other conscious activities, do not truly awaken your Kundalini, but they do help to release your resistance. That is the reason why this mindful activity is effective. The same effect can be obtained by meditating in a specific manner.

If you practice yoga in specific ways, you will be able to release resistance. Applying this Kundalini technique in the modern world is a major issue. Kundalini practices cannot evolve because so many people practice them incorrectly. They do not strive to overcome the underlying reluctance and make the necessary changes to live fully. Instead, they attempt to use Kundalini techniques in the same way that a boat sinks due to a large hole in the bottom of the boat. Even if you empty a bucket of water from the boat's deck every minute, the boat will only stay afloat for a short time because you are not addressing the underlying cause, which is the hole itself.

Most individuals address their Kundalini in this manner. They avoid the problem and try to conduct activities like yoga instead. It's pointless to engage in Kundalini-related activities unless you speak up, communicate your sincerity, and allow your entire force to enter your body.

So, attempt to dispel the myth that Kundalini is constantly awake and in a state of vitality. Nothing is more vital than your Kundalini energy or life force for being true to yourself. Everyone enters this world as a unique representation of self-consciousness. This implies that each individual enters this world with a unique essence, purpose, ideas, feelings, wants, needs, and functions in the cosmos. Our lives are marked by the development of one's genuine expression.

Awakening is synonymous with entering a state of complete honesty. Authenticity is part two of Awakening, regardless of which path you take. You must be aware of who you are. You are more than your physical body here on Earth. You can only be authentic to the extent that you are currently aware of yourself. This implies that you can only be authentic if you are self-aware.

Most of us are so discouraged and sad that we have no idea who we are. We are not conscious of our existence. What we are now is what will keep us secure in our environment and the social groupings that we have built. As a result, we may become carbon copies of others.

All of this happens to create resistance in you and cause you to deny yourself physically and spiritually. This will impact your desires, unique requirements, and truth, causing your Kundalini to be rejected. Opposing your Kundalini depletes your energy and, as a result, causes you to die. Nothing fosters Kundalini more than genuine inspiration fueling action; this is what living out your life is all about.

Kundalini Awakening is a phenomenon that some people encounter. Kundalini Awakening now entails removing one's resistance, allowing one to become fully embodied and filled with life force energy. In a second, they can be in sync with the essence.

Let's say someone visits a Kundalini meditation center and tries to incorporate it into their life. In that case, it will be difficult. They will be returned to the state of resistance because they have made no actual changes in their life.

In other words, when they are attempting to increase the process of allowing their Kundalini and the awareness that comes with it, and life does not reflect their authentic truth, they have problems and try to return to that state of being. It becomes unbearable to think about those thoughts and actions, let alone live that life.

Many people call this the "Kundalini syndrome." If you awaken, you will change how you interact with your surroundings. Increased sensitivity is a critical component of the Kundalini Awakening. It is the source of the disunity between the two states of being. It'll feel like you're trying to strangle yourself most of the time because there's a big gap, and you will feel excruciating dizziness.

So, if you have the Kundalini syndrome, you are likely to experience the symptoms associated with whichever element of your life you had previously experienced the most resistance in. If it occurs mentally, you will feel more significant psychological symptoms. If it was on a physical level, you would have more physical effects.

From a global standpoint, the awareness that arises due to Kundalini Awakening is a beautiful thing. It is not due to an excess of energy in the body. Kundalini is a new phenomenon, with little concept of how to adapt to modify one's life due to that sensitivity. It's the same as having consciousness but having no clue how to combine it with a world that operates at a continual level of unconsciousness.

Some of the things you used to accept could only be endured today because you numbed yourself to them. You could accomplish half of the things you believed you couldn't because you were in the state of resistance you were used to. You were doing half of the things you were doing because you didn't realize how bad they were. Maybe you've noticed yourself eating something bad for your body, but you still don't stop eating it.

To acclimate to most of the things you were exposed to, you had to go against your life force energy. Thus, you must truly adjust your life to that realization. The Kundalini Awakening makes this bearable. Being accustomed to a profoundly dysfunctional situation is not a sign of good health. All of the problems that most people experience have been caused by their attempts to reduce Kundalini energy rather than alter their awareness and do what they want to do.

It's not about Kundalini; it is about resistance to life force energy. If you've been on the path of Awakening for a long time, you're probably used to the discomfort of change and integration. You won't have Kundalini syndrome if you've matured to the point where you're accustomed to the holding state for this painful growth. Even if you experience some signs of change in awareness, it will not stabilize you. On the contrary, it will destabilize you if you haven't been on the road of Awakening for a long time and aren't used to pushing yourself to integrate opposites.

Assume you are not used to changing your behavior in response to the unavoidable instability of an uncertain universe or changing your Mutability, which is the foundation of who you are. In that case, you are likely to suffer from the Awakening process, especially if it is a sudden and unexpected shift in consciousness.

Keep in mind that the more you practice this Awakening, which can be painful, the simpler it will be for you to transform your consciousness. The higher your frequency shifts, the more your awareness moves. The closer your consciousness gets to where you are, the less probable that a shift in consciousness will take you to different conditions.

As we work toward our awakening, it is good to surround ourselves with one or more spiritual teachers who have been on the road for a while. A spiritual teacher is an example of someone who can coach you through the process or help you integrate it after it has occurred.

Kundalini Awakening is no different from any other type of spiritual Awakening. The Kundalini is the opposing power to the ego's extremely destructive expression. Awakening may be described as an incarnated form, and Kundalini practices are specific methods that permit that Awakening.

Kundalini yoga is also known as "consciousness yoga." It is a physical as well as a mental activity. Kundalini exercises are specific, repeated, and prescribed. In Kundalini yoga, you chant while working with your breath to raise your conscious awareness. It is a step toward reaching the summit of Awakening.

Kundalini is a life force energy, not a supernatural power in our existence. As a result, it is up to you whether you will resist or not.

CHAPTER 1: KUNDALINI HISTORY

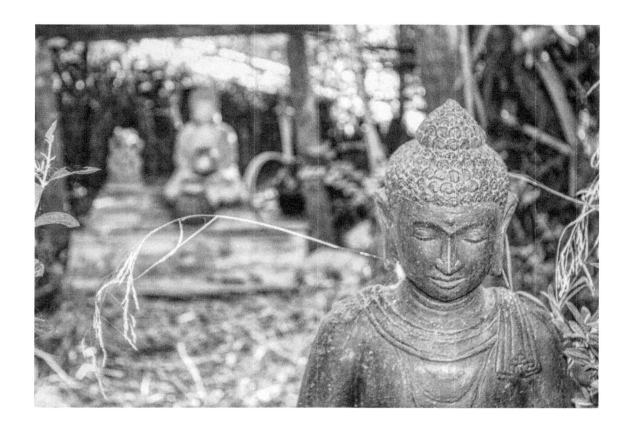

Although Hinduism and Buddhism are the two primary faiths commonly linked with the Kundalini Awakening, some practitioners claim that the awakening was present in Eastern religious traditions before their arrival.

The Upanishads, which date between 1,000 and 500 B.C., include the oldest reference of the Kundalini Awakening in literature. These publications depict Kundalini seminars where gurus sat with their followers and delivered spiritual teachings. Due to these teachers' visions and teachings, Kundalini Yoga evolved.

Kundalini Yoga was not taught to just anybody in the beginning. Years of rigorous initiation are required before mastering it. It was kept concealed from the general public for thousands of years, and Kundalini masters would only teach it to a few carefully selected disciples.

This gradually changed when professors opted to share material with the broader public, and researchers acquired access to previously restricted knowledge.

Sir John Woodroffe, Carl Jung, George King, Sri Aurobindo, Gopi Krishna, Tommaso Palamidessi, Julius Evola, Aleister Crowley, and Paramahansa Yogananda are among those who introduced Kundalini knowledge to the West.

To mention a few more, Yogananda, Yogi Bhajan, and Samael Aun Weor published books and have given courses about their Kundalini perspective.

Kundalini knowledge is now widely available and easily accessible via the internet, books, and classes. This might be because humanity is rapidly developing, and dispersed information will aid in guiding that evolution.

What is Kundalini Awakening?

Kundalini is an intense energy that coils around the base of the spine. The term is derived from the Sanskrit words "Kund" (to burn) and "Kunda" (to the coil). It is a major aspect of many faiths, including Hinduism and Buddhism, Jainism and Sikhism, and other current and historical belief systems.

It is thought that Kundalini activation offers enormous strength and spiritual enlightenment. As a result, several religions have developed techniques to activate this force. Some of these will be covered in this book.

The Kundalini is typically dormant in most of the population, although it may occasionally get activated purposely or inadvertently. When this happens, the energy ascends the spine until it reaches the top of the skull. It is stated that doing so connects one's energy to the rest of the universe.

When the Kundalini awakens, it may manifest as currents, sparks, waves, shocks, flames, winds, or flashes. This awakening can have beneficial and harmful consequences depending on how prepared a person is.

When a person reaches a particular level of spiritual growth, the Kundalini may arise independently. This timely awakening gives numerous benefits to the individual, which they might utilize to serve others.

However, there are times when it awakens early due to accidents, harsh events, or other causes. When this occurs, the individual may have adverse experiences.

The Kundalini's negative consequences result from anything impeding its journey to the skull. These obstructions might be produced by one or more of the following:

- Unclean body
- Negative energy
- Sustained thoughts and/or feelings
- Psychological trauma
- Unresolved problems
- Rigid beliefs
- Skepticism

Kundalini's Awakening rituals are intended to remove these impediments to activate the energy and clear its path to the top of the head.

Kundalini Awakening Indicators

Kundalini impacts both an individual's body and psyche. The following are some indicators of awakening:

- Shaking or twitching (involuntary motions)
- Unintentional body placement into "asanas" and hand positioning into "mudras"
- Unknown causes of heat, cold, vibrations, electric shocks, or tingling sensations
- Aches and pains
- Exceptional sensitivity to sensory stimuli, such as lights and noises
- Excessive emotional outbursts
- Apathy
- Inability to help
- An increased or decreased sexual desire
- Hallucinations
- Antisocial conduct
- Appetite Modifications
- Illnesses
- Irregular heartbeats
- High blood pressure
- Insomnia or sleepiness

These unpleasant sensations result from the energy disturbing the body's normal physical and energetic processes. They are not always penalties for awakening the Kundalini.

Fortunately, these effects are transitory and disappear as the individual's systems acclimatize to the new energy. This book will also provide advice on dealing with the adverse effects of the Kundalini Awakening.

Advantages of Kundalini Awakening

Many practitioners think that Kundalini activation leads to spiritual enlightenment. But what precisely does this mean?

Practitioners use the phrase "spiritual enlightenment" to denote a wide range of experiences. However, in Eastern faiths, enlightenment refers to a stage of human maturation that transforms how a person views life. Those who have experienced it describe it as being one with the universe and seeing through the veil of illusion to what is genuine.

When a person achieves enlightenment, their experience is real; they are not a phony individual becoming a genuine one – instead, they realize what they have always been. They encounter their true nature, buried beneath their incomplete perception of themselves.

The mind continuously projects reality; the objects in mind are only mirrors of what is truly real. The experience of enlightenment is experiencing things as they are. It is the point when the knower and the known become the same.

In enlightenment, the mind ceases to churn away thoughts and instead dwells on itself to know itself. Concerns and habits no longer distract the consciousness.

According to the Buddha, the mind is like a pool of water, with unpleasant emotions churning and muddying it. When it stops, the pool clears, making it easier to perceive reality.

Your mental clarity will allow you to look beyond illusions and straight at what is truly happening. This will clear up any uncertainty and assist you in breaking through patterns that most people are unaware of. This might also help you produce fresh ideas.

Kundalini links you to God and lifts your troubles. This results in a form of joy; not a fleeting kind, but something that may last your entire life. It promotes emotional stability and tranquility. It provides insight and awareness, allowing you to deal with events and people more effectively.

You will gain spiritual strength as a result of tuning in to the energy of the universe, which may result in any of the following: increased mental abilities, extrasensory perception (ESP), the ability to influence reality and other beings through your will, stronger physical prowess, faster healing and recovery from illness, patience, inspiration, determination, courage, and more. You will grow in various ways and inspire others to flourish as well.

Expanding your energy implies that you are experiencing your life to the fullest. As a consequence, you will get new experiences and chances. It will also boost your charm and capacity to inspire people.

Interacting with a spiritually enlightened individual produces the following results:

- Developing a nonjudgmental attitude
- Being composed
- Acquiring clarity
- Gaining an understanding of the purpose and meaning of life
- Increasing bravery
- Becoming at ease with uncertainty
- Having more self-assurance
- Becoming more accepting
- Increasing optimism

- Developing a relationship with one's inner self

The signs listed above indicate that you are in the presence of an awakened individual. Similarly, when you awaken, you will have these effects on others.

When you have successfully activated your Kundalini, you may realize that you will be able to perform things that you ordinarily could not or that most people cannot. This is why it used to be a highly kept secret, given only to those judged worthy of it.

You may realize that utilizing your abilities to damage another creature becomes more difficult as you gain insight into the other's predicament. You will be aware that you and your adversary are linked; you might even claim that you and the other person are the same creatures inhabiting separate bodies. It is still possible and typically easy to let go of anger after you have attained a certain degree of awareness.

How Kundalini can Help You

The practice of Kundalini Awakening is utilized to treat every sort of sickness. Whatever the reason, spiritual energy may always aid somehow, even if it is simply restoring hope to a life that has lost everything.

We can open our minds and see what was previously unseen to us via spiritual meditation. Meditation allows us to perceive the potential in others and the spiritual potential inside ourselves.

Allow our life energy to guide us on our journey, as Kundalini will not disappoint us. Life will begin to fall into place once we are entirely in sync with and with our Kundalini. We are constantly sending out energies into the world and drawing things back to ourselves. Things don't always come back right, but we can learn to regulate that. That is the Kundalini way: We get what we give. We draw things to us with our newfound awareness, and then use them to our benefit.

A Kundalini Awakening can cause physical symptoms such as tremors, laughter, sobbing, and even a burst of energy. As Kundalini travels down the Nadis (According to yoga theory, nadis carry life force energy), it is common to have side effects relating to the chakra through which Kundalini is attempting to go.

These may manifest as symptoms of emotional distress. The root chakra, for example, is concerned with one's security. We may feel vulnerable or insignificant when attempting to break through this obstacle because it is the exact sentiments that are causing the block in the first place. Kundalini will lead us through these difficulties and assist us in breaking down the barriers that are impeding the flow of the Nadis.

It is critical to comprehend what a Kundalini Awakening implies. Anyone and everyone can experience awakening, but it takes time and effort. It is vital not to go back into old habits following an incredible encounter. We may attempt to reproduce this technique or specific meditation session to recreate the experience, resulting in a halt in progress as our imagination begins to disrupt and replace our healing.

Our Nadis is a conduit for twelve chakras. Each one has a unique difficulty that obstructs Kundalini's path. Again, each person's experience will be unique because everyone has universal traumas and problems that they must overcome. We may obtain a far better physical and emotional state if we are to effectively break down these barriers.

The first chakra is our root chakra; it is red and is placed in the hip area. This chakra is associated with our mental patience and has an in-body relationship with the adrenals. This obstruction is most usually caused by physical injury. These traumas might have been caused by childhood trauma or even a terrifying vehicle accident. Many types of PTSD that leave wounds in our psyche will build the dam, halting energy flow. Muladhara is the Sanskrit name for this chakra. It is also the starting point for Kundalini to uncoil.

Our second chakra, which is orange, is positioned in the abdomen. This energy is associated with our sexual energies, specifically the ovaries and testicles. The emotional impediment is frequently present on this second level, and the spiritual reward of our waking here is purity. If we allow Kundalini to guide us, it will take us along the road of healing, allowing our emotional wounds to disappear. Svadhisthana is the Sanskrit word for our second chakra.

The third chakra, Manipura, is in our solar plexus and has a brilliant yellow color. The physical manifestations of this obstruction are frequently seen in the pancreas, and the primary culprit is our thinking. Kundalini's gift to us from this waking will be brightness. This may be a challenging stage for some to conquer, but the obstruction may be eliminated with the correct Kundalini yoga techniques.

Our green chakra is the fourth. This energy is centered in the heart and is associated with physical ramifications there. Relationships are the source of the problems that wreak havoc on our emotions. This includes not just romantic ties but also family and friend relationships. Our fourth chakra serves as a balanced focus for our energy. Cleansing this chakra might result in a change from "me to us."

In Sanskrit, the fifth chakra is called Vishudda, emitting a deep blue light. This chakra is located in the throat and is associated with communication concerns. Unspoken words will poison us from within our bodily being. Maintaining effective communications is critical, although it may take some time to master. Chatting someone's ear off for an hour is different from sitting down and making sure we connect and get our point through. Some of us may be waiting for someone to apologize or vice versa. Most of the time, the chance is missed due to a misunderstanding in or a lack of communication. For this specific obstruction, physical qualities for the fifth chakra will dwell within the thyroid. Kundalini, if cleansed, will give us the gift of togetherness.

The sixth chakra is positioned near the forehead and is purple. This chakra's Sanskrit name is Ajna, and its physical manifestation is in the pituitary gland. Our eyesight impedes Kundalini's ascension to this level. Once we've broken past this impenetrable barrier, the most frequent accomplishment is the authority over our lives.

Our seventh awakening is located in the white chakra of the head, which is known as Sahasrara in Sanskrit. This link is with our pineal gland and is obstructed by spiritual issues. When we reach this state of waking, the most typical outcome is a heightened level of consciousness.

The eighth chakra is a deep dark energy field that emanates above the head. This energy is physically connected to our thymus gland and signifies our ability to move forward and initiate a flow of transformation. Reaching this awareness stage can result in a shamanic awakening, allowing one to project onto multiple astral realms and travel in their dreams. Blockages in this chakra are frequently associated with karma and even losing loved ones.

The ninth chakra is our golden chakra, an arm's length above the head. This energy's physical characteristics are frequently linked to the diaphragm. Awakening this level will, in some ways, open a higher sense of empathy. We should be able to detect the "DNA" of other people's souls. This talent will also aid us in achieving peace by allowing us to open our souls and give back to the land.

The tenth chakra is brown and is located about a foot and a half underground. This energy keeps us grounded and gives us a feeling of pragmatism. This chakra is associated with our bones. It provides us with a greater feeling of grounding and our heritage to the soil. It is critical to be able to ground oneself, especially while trying to meditate or recuperate after a traumatic situation.

The eleventh chakra is a rose-colored energy field surrounding our torso, hands, and feet. After this awakening, Kundalini may assist us in shifting supernatural and natural forces, and it may even provide us with a sense of leadership and competence. This chakra will physically connect to the connective tissue of the body.

Finally, the twelfth and last chakra encircles our complete auric field. This chakra has no color and instead emits dazzling energy. This energy is linked to 32 in-body connections. This stumbling obstacle will always be unique to each individual. Our twelfth aura reflects our unique and spiritual journey, and the gift of Kundalini Awakening will be individualized to each individual.

When we master our Kundalini Awakening, we change our entire perspective on the world. This change should improve our spirits and provide us tranquility of mind and body.

Those who suffer from depression, anxiety, or post-traumatic stress disorder may find it more difficult to remove the impediments to Kundalini's flow. Many of these traumas will cause us to "lock" these gates, causing our energy to be stifled. It will take a lot more practice, but removing those impediments can save our lives. When we don't know how to utilize our minds, they may be harmful, but Kundalini can assist in ensuring that no damage comes to us if we know how to ask for guidance.

Some of us may have previously had one or more Kundalini Awakenings without even realizing it. Anything may cause these breakthroughs in our energies: a near-death experience, a therapy session, or even a sporting event. If it has meaning for the human, our Divine energy will respond.

The act of Pranayama, or breathing practice, is the first and most crucial thing to master on our path to waking. The first Pranayama practice we'll look at is Nadi Shodhana (breathing practice), which translates to "channel cleansing." We may automatically relax and enter a contemplative state by doing breathing techniques. This exercise will also help relax our spine, open up our channels, and allow Kundalini to begin her journey through our Sushumna Nadi.

We'll talk about various forms of energy and what meditations we should start with. These practices are only the beginning of our spiritual awakening, so we must be open and prepared for an entirely new world. All of our activities will begin basic and brief to introduce Kundalini Yoga exercises into our lives in a way that does not overwhelm or stress us. This is not to say that we should stop meditating; it depends on the individual and how much they can accomplish comfortably. It is always beneficial to push ourselves, but we might halt our growth by doing too much at once, stifling the uncoiling of our Kundalini.

CHAPTER 2: KUNDALINI'S CONNECTION TO PRANA AND THE CHAKRAS

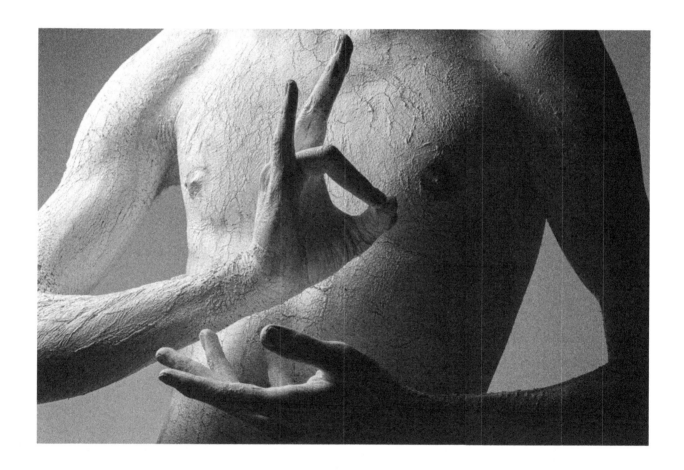

Energy Secret Yoga

In Kundalini yoga, we learn how to increase our energy, synchronize the impulses of our nervous system, eliminate energetic blockages, regulate our hormones, and raise our mood to enable the pure light of our genuine self to show through. While other types of yoga concentrate on physical postures, Kundalini yoga focuses on how the postures affect our energy and mindset. Postures, movement, breathing, meditation, mantras, and lifestyle create extraordinary personal energy shifts. Kundalini is the focused life energy that unlocks our potential. It is a latent energy that urges us to be awakened within – permeating us when activated, energizing our cells, bringing health and vigor, and connecting our awareness to the limitless. Kundalini yoga practices have evolved over thousands of years. They are potent instruments for opening up our energy pathways so that the proper quantity of energy at the right frequency may flow effortlessly through our entire bodies.

Kundalini yoga is based on the idea that our physical body and energy are inextricably linked. What we do with our bodies has a corresponding influence on our energy, and what we do with our energy has a corresponding effect on our bodies. Tightness in our hamstrings, for example, is an obstruction in the energy that would typically move through that portion of our body. That tightness is referred to as opacity because it prevents the passage of interior light. We may release the equivalent blocked-up energy by using ancient Kundalini yoga practices to stretch the muscle or move a limb via the energy field that surrounds our body. Our inner light might then begin to pour into previously confined areas. The consequent impact on our body and psyche is tremendous. Not only does the muscle become more supple, but our consciousness alters, our mind clears, and the new energy improves our genetic functioning. As light passes through our energy field, our consciousness awakens. Our energy level surges, and we feel alive and hopeful, like a flower bursting from the soil after a long, hard winter.

For thousands of years, Kundalini yoga was kept secret in India, taught exclusively to devout disciples who were judged worthy. Yogi Bhajan went to the United States from his native India in the 1960s. He began teaching Kundalini yoga as a self-improvement method, and it immediately became popular. He wrote over thirty books and traveled extensively, teaching Kundalini yoga worldwide until his death in 2004. The writers have spent a significant amount of time studying Kundalini yoga. We have sourced the exercises in this book for historical authenticity, so you can identify whether Yogi Bhajan gave an exercise, is a classic from the past, or is a visualization we present to clarify a concept.

Kundalini Spirit

Kundalini's yoga practice frequently results in a natural experience of oneness with global energy bigger than our limited sense of self. However, Kundalini yoga is not a religion and may be performed by anybody with any spiritual belief. It also does not require any specific spiritual concept. Whether you belong to a formal religion or not, it is common for actions to boost one's sentiments of spirituality. When the amazing stream of our energy is finally allowed to come through the layers of shielding we have put up all our lives, flashes of understanding, cosmic breakthroughs, tears of delight, and signs of surrender are regular occurrences. We encourage you to surrender to the gift of a spiritual experience rather than opposing it out of fear. In reality, it is past time to let go of your apprehension about your brilliance. To express the oneness of universal spirit in Kundalini yoga, we utilize the phrases God, the infinite, spirit source, and the universe throughout this text. However, they are only phrases, and you are invited to take the spirit that works for you from this book and leave the rest behind.

Prana Energy

When discussing Kundalini's awakening, Prana will be referenced frequently. In yoga, Prana refers to the life energy that permeates everything and everyone. Even modern scientists are beginning to accept this. People assumed that everything was merely a collection of molecules and atoms for many years. When they looked closer at buildings, they realized that they were composed of energy. This indicates that nothing can exist without Prana. That is why you must comprehend and employ Prana.

When you meditate, you fuel your body with Prana. Kirlian photography, a type of photography that allows you to view people's energy and aura, was utilized by researchers to demonstrate this claim. That is why meditation is so beneficial. The incredible thing is that the power of personal energy isn't new, but people are only now becoming aware of it.

Personal Prana is the Prana that lives within you, while global Prana is the Prana that exists globally. Both sources are accessible and can be used at any time. Most gurus would tell you that employing personal Prana is inefficient since it physically drains you. As a result, it is ideal for tapping into universal energy if you need to consume a lot of energy.

We'll look at how to regulate and use Prana to help you comprehend it better. You will be able to feel it as a result of this.

Prana Control

The first thing you should understand about Prana before managing it is that it follows thinking. Using your thoughts to control Prana is one of the most powerful methods. How do you utilize your intellect to do this? Visualization is the key. Visualization is frequently associated with the sense of sight. While this is true, you may improve your visualization skills by activating all of your senses. When you attempt to imagine a dog, you not only see it but also feel it, hear it, and smell it. It is critical to employ your sense of feeling when dealing with Prana. You want to be able to sense the energy as it moves. You may effortlessly regulate Prana by simply using your sense of touch. This is referred to as tactile visualization.

Enough philosophizing; let us now look at how to govern Prana. This initial exercise is only a vision, but it will assist you in becoming acquainted with Prana.

Begin By Relaxing and Focusing on Your Hand

Begin to feel and sense your particular Prana flowing through you now. Visualize your Prana accumulating in your palm. Feel the buildup of energy.

You will find your energy collecting in that hand as you practice. Remember to employ as many of your senses as possible. This will be a lot easier than it appears once you get started. You must remain focused on what you are attempting to accomplish while performing this activity. Thoughts such as "my mind is playing tricks on me" may enter your mind. You must force these out. That's your skepticism speaking. If you do this regularly, you will soon be able to manage your Prana.

Another Fundamental Exercise

Rub your hands together until you feel a warm sensation in your palms.

Put your hands in front of you as if holding a baseball. Visualize yourself drawing universal Prana into the ball you're holding in your hands.

Prana can take on any shape, so you may imagine it in any manner you desire. Think of it as white light. Keep an eye on it as it travels and accumulates in the area between your palms.

Can you sense it? Concentrate your thoughts and attention on it and let your visualization take control. Allow yourself to be receptive to sensations and relax, allowing universal energy to flow through you.

After you've mastered these fundamental Prana exercises, you'll discover how simple it is to manipulate and use Prana. You will be able to employ Prana in many ways as you become more familiar with it.

Prana Vibration

Prana is the energy that runs through us, keeping us alive, igniting our lives, and allowing us to shine. Prana has a captivating charm, a charisma all its own. When Prana runs freely and unobstructed through our bodies, we may be radiantly healthy and reach our greatest potential. Our Prana is, in many ways, who we are. If we could capture our energy in a photograph, it would be a bright, three-dimensional mandala of vibrating frequencies and harmonies resonating through our bodies and the electromagnetic field surrounding us.

Our breath is the primary means of transporting pranic energy to each cell and into the electromagnetic field that encompasses our bodies. We may also offer and receive Prana from other people, animals, and plants via touch, prayer, and relationships. Even a hug generates a Prana exchange. Prana enters our bodies through our diet and is absorbed through our skin. When we fall in love and think of our beloved, and they think about us, we exchange pranic energy in one of the most beautiful ways.

Kundalini is the human body's concentrated form of Prana. It is the divine force within the human. Kundalini rests at the base of the spine until the frequency necessary for activation is attained and obstacles in our energy pathways are eliminated. It rises through the central channel of the spine to ignite our life force. When the Kundalini energy is activated, it causes a spectacular chain of events to occur in the mind and body. The awakening incorporates the soul's vitality with the tangible realities of existence. It may appear to be a mysterious procedure, but it is only a question of realizing your potential. We'll keep things as straightforward and uncomplicated as possible.

A sphere of energy surrounds our bodies and vibrates with the bioactivity occurring within us. This field, known as the electromagnetic field or the aura — words that will be used interchangeably throughout the book — is where transformation begins. Kundalini yoga techniques employ Prana to produce energy adjustments in our magnetic field to modify our cellular expression to one of health.

There ais a lot of talk these days about how our ideas create our world. This is correct; nonetheless, Prana is what fuels our thinking. The mind will not just reason its way out of locked patterns of dread. What we believe is whatever is set in action by the force of our Prana. Because our ideas are energetic wave patterns, we shift them with our Prana. Our Prana is responsible for the electromagnetic field's brightness and power by strengthening, energizing, healing, expanding, and purifying it.

Prana's Four Qualities

The four Prana properties listed below give a foundation for working with Kundalini energy.

The Drive to Activation

Regardless of our circumstances, we all have a calling that drives us to continue ahead in our lives. That calling is embedded in Prana, motivating us to grow. The cosmos wants us to awaken, and it will work with us in endless detail to help us become the healthiest, most luminous people we can be. When we set Prana in action, all sorts of events and synchronicities occur to aid in our waking.

We sense the calling and trust the support on a soul level, but we frequently hold ourselves back. We unconsciously dread re-creating mistakes from our past or being rejected by others, so we freeze and build an energy block to our activation. Those energy-stumbling obstacles become routine and intimidating. They may, however, be dispelled by altering the flow and frequency of our Prana. Once the inner obstacles have been removed, the light of our true selves can shine from the core of our being, through our bodies, and into the world around us. Prana has the power to unleash your radiance. It manifests as our desire for self-actualization, as our soul longs to complete its mission.

Frequency

Everything vibrates at a low level of frequency. The greater your frequency, the stronger your magnetic force. Our Prana frequency is the key to our health, consciousness, and attracting force. Within each of us is an energetic combination of pleasure and sadness, joys and challenges, hopes and dreams; we are a vibrating, three-dimensional mandala of our unique self. We are constantly communicating our energy to the rest of the planet.

Our mood determines how we perceive the vibration of our Prana. Our Prana constantly sends a personality portrait, and we can learn to change the frequency to one of health and attractiveness. Love is the enigmatic vibration that expands our minds, ignites our health, and awakens our potential. It unlocks shutters that would otherwise remain closed, allowing the light of our spirit to shine through the dazzling diamond of our existence. It is not always easy to change our frequency. We get enslaved to our typical emotional patterns. We may, however, alter the vibratory frequency of our energy back to its source — love — via Kundalini yoga techniques. Then, a torrent of extraordinary benefits — emotional, physical, and spiritual — flows forth.

Resonance

To live a life in harmony with your actual nature, you need to learn about the scientific phenomenon called sympathetic resonance. Our inner frequency radiates from our physical body into the electromagnetic environment surrounding us. Our resonance increases and harmonizes with other people's frequencies all across the planet. Suppose your electromagnetic field is vibrating with thankfulness energy, for example. That vibration will echo with comparable frequencies in every location your electromagnetic field effects, whether within your body or in the actual environment. This is how our ideas make our existence a reality. Our ideas produce a vibration that resonates with and activates the same character we are emitting. That is why moving out of chronic harmful thought patterns is so important. One of the benefits of Kundalini yoga is the ability to do this.

Your real brilliance and inspirations may be beneficial, if channeled, since they draw others of the same frequency into your life. Remember, like attracts like.

Radiance

Our glitter and shine are defined by radiance. It is the light released by our energy frequencies, fueled by Prana. Our light resonates across the aura, connecting us to the limitless. We become magnetic creatures that attract chances and achievement via synchronicity rather than effort when we have a healthy glow. Our radiant body's energy begins with the spin of atoms within our cells and extends to the ends of the cosmos. We may connect with the highest potential of our existence and attract love, peace, and grace by aligning that atomic spin with our soul's mission and removing the barriers and fears that impede our energy flow. Our whole energy field has the potential for brilliance.

Golden Light Breath for Prana Activation

The constant and magnetic flow of life energy is connected via the Golden Light Breath. We advise reclining the steps below while lying. Still, you may use this breathing method to tune in to your Prana anywhere — at your desk, while walking, or sitting motionless in meditation. This is a fantastic technique to undertake before falling asleep when lying down in bed.

1. Place your hands on your lower tummy while lying on your back. Envision your breath as a golden light instead of invisible air as you inhale and exhale.
2. Inhale deeply and allow your abdomen to expand like a balloon. Slow your breathing as deeply and slowly as possible while seeing your tummy expand. Consider your breath to be formed of golden light. On the inhale, fill every part of your lungs.
3. Allow the golden light to flow through your entire body and into the field outside your skin while holding your breath.
4. Allow your tummy to deflate as you exhale so your belly button pulls toward your spine. Feel the golden light stretching over your skin and into the space around you, mixing with the brightness of the cosmos.

5. Exhale for a few seconds before slowly and deliberately inhaling again. Continue to inhale and exhale deeply and slowly, with a soft hold at either end of the breath, envisioning the breath as golden light.

6. Feel a large global pool of love enter your being, pouring through your nose, filling your lungs, and circulating throughout your body, loving you and nurturing your cells.

7. Continue to breathe slowly and deeply for three to eleven minutes, holding your breath after each inhale and exhale. With each inhale, feel this light and knowledge pushing into you and vibrating throughout your aura as you hold your breath, loving you, nurturing you, and washing away stress. Imagine letting go of everything preventing you from igniting your brilliance as you exhale.

8. Finally, examine and accept your feelings. After practicing this breath, you may have a profoundly pleasant experience or encounter resistance and dissatisfaction. Whatever you're experiencing is important; don't attempt to change it. Allow the sensations to come and go as they please.

The Phenomenon of Love Frequency

We are more than our physical bodies; we are our energy. Being filled to overflowing with cheerful, robust vitality is the natural result of having our energy resonate at the frequency of love. This is the condition of being at our core. In the biological environment of love, our DNA expresses itself ideally in ways we had no idea were conceivable. We get fresh awareness and intuition. We have a deeper connection with people because we know that the same love in their souls also resonates in ours. We discover that we can channel an unbelievable quantity of bright energy into our bodies and lives. Life falls in love with us, and we fall in love with it. This is a wonder.

When we vibrate at a loving frequency, our external world alters, and we become magnets for igniting our potential. When the enticing force of love fills our body and is projected into our aura, it's as though what we genuinely desire — our true potential — seeks us out. This is why the name Love Frequency Phenomenon was developed.

Love is a human experience of the universe's most powerful physical force. We experience the attraction force that keeps atoms together when we sense love. This energizing power also binds people together. It energizes our physical body, promotes cell health, and shines through our spirit. Rather than looking for it elsewhere, we discover it most easily within ourselves. Kundalini yoga can assist us in accessing the love frequency phenomena by removing the boundaries that prevent our gifts from shining brightly in the world. Love is a vibration that can make the impossible possible.

Prana's Transition from Fear to Love

We may believe that turning off our lights would allow more love into our lives or would benefit people around us. We conceal to enable others to shine, and then we are wounded and disappointed when they do not give us the affection we desire. We give away our light to satisfy others and accept it as a natural part of life.

There is a soul journey that cannot be postponed. It might begin as an inward tickle, the spirit within taunting us to be noticed. We strive to maintain a condition of numbness, but our soul eventually demands to be acknowledged, supported, and released.

You've felt the tickling sensation if you've picked up this book. We have a fantastic opportunity to shine. The earth requires each of our lights. It's something we're aware of. Now is the time to start walking in our light.

When the majesty of your own soul's light spreads, resistances dissolve, and life begins to flow. Synchronicities occur. A wisdom that will not harm anyone will emerge. This is your most powerful and natural state of existence. Thus, it is not acceptable to conceal your light.

The Nature

Prana, by definition, cannot be destroyed, yet it may be manipulated. This is why it is stated that everything is everlasting. Prana is not constrained by time or place. It has no boundaries and is limitless. Many people consider Prana to be God. Those who can control it have the potential to wield enormous power. However, to do so successfully, you must have a well-focused mind. Another reason meditation is essential is that it teaches you how to use your mind's power more efficiently.

Prana is extremely sensitive. The Prana will disappear if you lose attention. To control Prana, you must first manage your mind. But it isn't something you should worry about; it will come in time.

Healing Chakras

Because you require a healthy chakra system to activate your Kundalini, you must understand how to heal them. All of your chakras are inextricably linked to your physical body. Healthy chakras maintain your physical body in good shape. One of the simplest methods to maintain your chakras in a healthy way is to keep your body healthy and fit. This is why it is critical to exercise regularly. One of the most natural methods to purify your chakras is to exercise.

You also don't have to overdo it with your workouts. Simple exercises like walking or jogging are ideal. The essential thing is to love yourself and your body and let go of all bad energy.

Eating healthy is another crucial aspect of maintaining the health of your chakras. Make sure to eat lots of veggies and limit your intake of processed meals. Some people believe that you should also eliminate dairy and meat items. You do not have to be vegan but try to eat as many greens and nutritious meals as possible. If you aren't already a healthy eater, you may become one by progressively incorporating better meals and gradually removing harmful ones.

Making beneficial lifestyle adjustments is also essential. If you smoke, you should quit. You don't have to quit smoking cold turkey; lower the number of cigarettes you smoke each day until you reach zero. Also, if you are a big drinker, attempt to limit your intake of alcoholic beverages. The better your physical health, the more invigorated and clean your chakra system will be.

It is difficult to remain healthy, especially when you are accustomed to engaging in many bad practices. This does not have to be the case indefinitely. Be grateful that you were able to observe and learn from these practices. Begin with minor modifications and consider doing beneficial activities for your body. Some traditions place stringent regulations on their adherents. Some people go so far as to abstain from all animal products and alcohol to activate their Kundalini.

The excellent news is that, unless you follow a tradition that requires this, all you need to do is live a healthy lifestyle. It is equally critical to act in a good manner. It may be difficult at first to implement these adjustments, but they will quickly become second nature. You will eventually become engrossed with how great you feel due to your new healthy behaviors.

Healing Meditation

Aside from leading a healthy lifestyle, you may repair your chakras through meditation and yoga. All meditation activities will benefit your chakras. However, specific approaches are more focused on stimulating and purifying your chakras than others. The following approach will assist you in clearing and energizing your chakras. This may be done daily or if you feel your systems are out of balance. If you've been exposed to negativity, this is a terrific method to detoxify yourself and feel more energized.

This meditation will travel through each chakra and charge it with the color that corresponds to it. We'll work our way through your chakras, starting with your root chakra and ending with your crown chakra.

- Take a comfortable and calm meditation posture.
- Allow yourself to relax and take a few deep, soft breaths in and out.
- Pay attention to your root chakra. This will serve as your basis. Consider a crimson ball of light entering from the astral dimension and passing into your head chakra. Allow it to go all the way to the base of your spine, where your root chakra is located. Feel the chakra's properties become more powerful. Consider how this red light may energize and cleanse your root chakra. The more energy sent toward this chakra, the stronger it will become. Allow this light to energize your chakra until you feel focused and anchored.
- When you're ready, you'll start charging your second chakra. Consider transforming a red ball of light into an orange ball of light. Allow this ball of light to enter your sacral chakra, just below your belly button. Allow this orange ball of light to revitalize and purify your chakra. Feel that the chakra's traits and qualities become energized as this ball of light energizes your sacral chakra. Don't rush through this. Repeat this process until you are sure that your chakra has absorbed all of the energy it requires. But be careful not to absorb too much. If you begin to feel uneasy, it is time to go on.
- Once you've done charging your sacral chakra, notice how the orange ball of light changes to a yellow ball of light. Allow this light to move up to your solar plexus chakra, located above your belly button.

Allow this light ball to invigorate your solar plexus chakra, absorbing as much energy as it needs. Feel as though all of the traits linked with this chakra become more powerful. Move on to the next chakra after you feel it has been fully healed.

- Notice how the yellow ball of light changes into a green ball of light. Allow this light to move up to your heart chakra, located in the center of your chest. Feel the abundance of love that this light sends into your chakra. Sit with this ball of light in your heart chakra and let it fully charge and cleanse the chakra. Allow it to absorb as much energy as it needs and watch as the traits become more powerful. Move on to the next step when you're ready.

- Notice how the green ball of light changes into a blue ball of light. Allow it to make its way to your throat chakra. Feel your throat chakra grow more potent. Allow your chakra to absorb all of the energy it needs. Allow this ball of light to continue to restore your chakra. Move on to the next step when you're ready.

- Let the blue ball of light turn into an indigo glow. Allow this light to pass through your Third Eye (In 6th Chakra you will learn in detail about third eye). As the light cleanses and restores your Third Eye, feel your intuition grow more powerful. Allow your chakra to absorb as much energy as it needs from the ball of light. When you're ready, proceed to the final chakra.

- Keep an eye on the indigo ball of light as it transforms into a purple ball of light. This ball of light ascends to your head chakra. Allow this light to charge and strengthen your chakra. Allow it to absorb as much energy from this purple spinning ball of light as it needs. When you feel your head chakra is cleansed, release this blazing ball of light.

- Visualize the purple glowing light fading away and returning to the astral world.

- Visualize all of your chakras at once and pay attention to how energetic and cleansed they are. Take note of how they sparkle and glitter in their unique lights. Take note of how you feel joyful, purified, and empowered.

- Gradually return your focus to your actual body. Wiggle your toes and fingers slowly before opening your eyes slowly.

You can devote as much time to each of your chakras during this meditation. Do not go to the next chakra until you are confident that it has been thoroughly charged and cleansed. You must maintain the characteristics of each chakra in mind while you move through this meditation. You will be able to identify when the chakra has been charged because you will feel those traits strengthen.

Imagine a white light activating each chakra if you find it difficult to see each hue at first. Once you've gotten used to working with your chakras, you'll find that employing the correct colors works better since they're more powerful. Because the colors of the chakras are the same, ROYGBIV, you may easily recall the colors of the chakras from root to crown by memorizing the rainbow. Most essential is that you enjoy the process and don't get too worked up over it.

Prana vs. Kundalini

Some individuals get the terms Kundalini and Prana mixed up. So, what exactly is Prana? Prana is defined as energy. Prana is thought to reside everywhere in spirituality. It is both inside and outside of you. Nothing can live in the absence of Prana. You will discover how to tap and harness Prana later in this book. You will be able to perform amazing things if you master Prana. This is because everything is formed from Prana. You will be a master of everything if you master the technique of controlling Prana. It should be mentioned that everything is comprised of energy, even things you can't see with your eyes (Prana).

Take notice that this energy is not the same as the energy found by Einstein. This energy, or Prana, is not constrained by any formula. It is and has infiltrated everything. Is the Kundalini the same as the Prana? No, it is not. Prana is a general phrase that refers to all energy, whereas Kundalini is more particular. Kundalini is the coiled snake at the base of your spine, yearning to be released. It should also be mentioned that this snake is ethereal — it is composed of Prana — rather than coarse material. Prana accepts everything. You are Prana, and everything around you is Prana as well.

Kundalini Energy and Your Chakras

Chakras are an essential part of most yoga practices. These power centers can be found at seven distinct spots on your body. If you are unfamiliar with chakras, we will go through them briefly in a moment. Kundalini has a tremendous and profound influence on each of your chakras due to its nature. Many waking people describe having a lot of energy in their chakras, which causes symptoms and sensations. Some of them are enjoyable, while others may be dubious or even alarming if you are inexperienced with the experience. We will look at how Kundalini affects your chakras, what to expect, and how to cope with these experiences.

The 7 Physical Chakras

1. Your body has seven physical energy centers that you would feel throughout your Kundalini Awakening. While each soul has numerous chakras, these seven chakras are related to the physical body. Each chakra has a distinct color, location, and function. These are their names:
2. The Root Chakra
3. The Sacral Chakra
4. The Solar Plexus Chakra
5. The Heart Chakra
6. The Throat Chakra
7. The Third Eye Chakra
8. The Crown Chakra

Let's look at how Kundalini's energy affects these chakras.

The Root Chakra and Kundalini

The root chakra, located at the base of your spine, is where Kundalini lies dormant until you activate it. When Kundalini wakes, it does not always indicate that the root chakra is also aroused. Typically, this chakra will have adequate energy to aid in awakening. However, until full Kundalini energy has extended throughout your chakra system, your chakras will not be awakened or altered.

When you awaken, you may feel tremendous vibrations in your root chakra. As you connect to this chakra and experience the energy flowing through it, you may find a strong affinity for the color red. Some people describe feeling firmly grounded in the Earth as this process begins.

The Sacral Chakra and Kundalini

Many people report feeling dark energy when Kundalini energy begins to flow via the sacral chakra. This is due to the sacral chakra's tendency to hang onto deep-seated difficulties that the person has been holding onto. This area will contain any traumas, whether inherited or acquired personally. As the energy awakens and stirs, they will be confronted with these traumas and given a conscious chance to become aware of and repair them. This may be pretty strong if you are still in the early stages of the Kundalini Awakening. This is frequently the cause of individuals holding back and erecting barriers and resistances. When this chakra is balanced and cleared, the energy contributes to feelings of calm, fearlessness, and strength of will.

The Solar Plexus Chakra and Kundalini

Because the solar plexus chakra is located in the middle of the body, we frequently have energy coming up from the Earth and down from the source. Many folks describe feeling chronic weariness when the awakened energy enters this place. Some people cannot get out of bed for extended periods. This is due to the sacral chakra's ability to quickly become overburdened with energy, causing it to drain from burnout. Taking the time to stabilize this energy and repair any damage to the energy fields in your solar plexus chakra can help alleviate these symptoms.

As the chakra completely wakes and manifests its power, you will realize that it creates a sense of oneness. People in this condition no longer feel isolated from the rest of the world but instead, they comprehend that we are all connected. This is often a watershed moment in a person's spiritual awakening, as their view on life and the world around them is forever altered.

The Heart Chakra and Kundalini

People are allowed to become aware of their emotional burdens and bring healing through the awakening of the heart chakra. Although the heart chakra is connected with creativity, love, compassion, and empathy, these may not be your first experiences when you awaken. Instead, you may experience depression, feeling overwhelmed, fear, frustration, guilt or shame, and disappointment. However, this will begin to clear, making room for the fully opened heart chakra's more priceless and tranquil experiences.

Many people who are in the process of waking their heart chakra may begin to hear noises from other dimensions. Angelic voices, beautiful music, and a keen awareness of the noises around them become commonplace. They also grow more sympathetic toward others around them, frequently sensing others' feelings. This sensitive chakra, when balanced, assists you in navigating your oneness with the world around you with an open heart and a loving goal.

The Throat Chakra and Kundalini

Kundalini enters the neck chakra and fills the cervical plexus behind the throat. This affects your throat, mouth, ears, and hearing. During this chakra awakening, you begin to understand the duality of light and darkness and bring consciousness to the opposites. You may become aware of your unbalanced throat chakra during the awakening process. Any organs connected with this chakra might be suffering from chronic illness, disease, or damage.

When the chakra is balanced and aroused, you will feel more honest and able to express yourself. It becomes easier to communicate with love and kindness when you stand firm in your boundaries. This chakra enjoys expressing itself through music, singing, speaking, chanting, and mantras.

The Third Eye Chakra and Kundalini

The pineal gland is associated with your Third Eye chakra, which is said to naturally shut down around ages 9 and 10 for the average person. This chakra is the command center for the whole subtle body system and your dealings with the metaphysical. When this chakra is blocked, it is difficult to feel the sensations linked with your clair senses. The clair senses are psychic skills associated with the five senses of tasting, seeing, feeling, hearing, and smelling. It can be difficult to connect with the world truly and thoroughly around you, and you may feel detached or disconnected from others, your higher self, and source awareness.

You may feel pressure in your Third Eye during the awakening process, have vivid dreams, and have regular clairvoyant experiences. As it awakens and begins to take in more than it is used to, it may seem overpowering or even out of control at first. Because this is the command center for your other clair senses, you may start to feel, hear, sense, and engage with the energies around you. This might be pretty overwhelming at first.

This chakra begins to support your ability to consciously connect to what most people are unconscious to as it balances. You become more accustomed to the energetic experiences you are having. Your clair senses become more stable, and you gain the capacity to connect easily and comfortably with the metaphysical world around you. This chakra is frequently responsible for bringing spiritual healing to the other chakras because it can bring awareness to the parts of you that require conscious attention for healing.

The Crown Chakra and Kundalini

The crown chakra is depicted in Kundalini by a thousand-petal lotus that opens out on top of your head. Some traditions think it is squarely on top of your head, while others say it is above your head. This chakra is in charge of assisting us in realizing that we know nothing and everything, and that we have merged with the completeness of everything that is.

When your crown chakra begins to awaken, you may feel various physical sensations on the top of your head. Many people describe irritation, vibration, burning, crawling, and other sensations in this region. As it wakes, you may get a mild to severe headache. When it is balanced, you will no longer have these experiences, and you will feel divinely linked to source energy at all times. This helps you to reintroduce energy and truth into your body.

How to Awaken Kundalini by Working with the Chakras

While some individuals choose to let the Kundalini energy awaken their chakras in their own time, others prefer to direct it in a precise order. Many Kundalini gurus and instructors would advise folks just starting on their Kundalini journey to begin with the crown chakra rather than the root chakra. The lower chakras are connected with darker, more subconscious energies. This can be difficult to confront for someone who has recently woken up and can be pretty traumatic if you are not supported by someone who understands what you are going through.

Furthermore, beginning with the crown chakra connects you to source energy and helps you progress into your Third Eye chakra, crucial in spiritual healing. This implies you can navigate through the remainder of the chakra system with the help of your Third Eye. This can significantly influence many people's capacity to assist meaningful, focused healing. Furthermore, it enables people to fully repair everything, rather than accidentally hanging onto specific things or extending the experience due to a lack of cognitive understanding of what has to be healed or why.

While you may take control and finish this using whichever ways you want, it is typically suggested to begin at the head chakra and work your way down. This may assist you in experiencing a more gradual awakening that is simpler to digest for your bodily self and egoic thinking. That way, you won't have deep and overwhelming resistance to waking, which might result in significant blockages that prevent you from experiencing the complete process.

CHAPTER 3: MAPS OF KUNDALINI'S DOMAIN

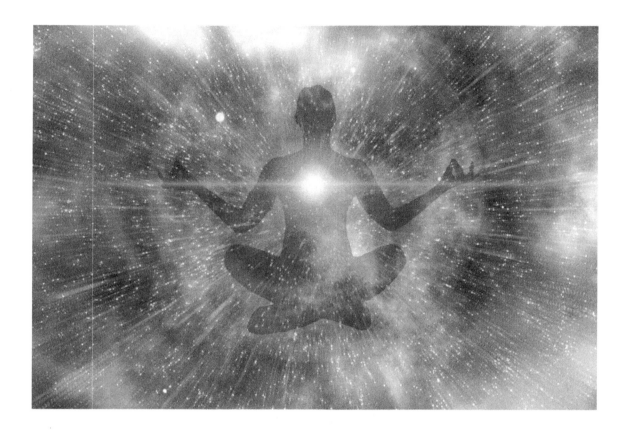

For thousands of years, the yogic tradition has investigated Kundalini's power of Awareness, mapping out the domains. She operates within the structures and dynamics of what emerges in the states of consciousness that manifest when Kundalini rises.

Kundalini transforms one from a state of being unaware of and separated from the Divine, as well as from the deep meaning and purpose of one's life, to a state of intimate knowledge of one's unity with the Divine, with everyone, and with the entire world, even while the mind and body function skillfully in the everyday world.

Living Sahaja Samadhi, or living meditation, is the ultimate objective of Kundalini unfolding, living in the inherent condition of being that has transcended and incorporated all domains of experience. Kundalini transforms the desires for love, pleasure, and freedom by revealing how they are finally satisfied by living in one's actual essence, embracing and being loved by the Infinite as oneself.

By providing maps of the spiritual landscape to be traveled on our soul's journey, the yogic tradition provides insightful accounts of how Kundalini's force functions. Maps are visual representations of reality. The ancient sages mapped and handed on to us the structure and dynamics of the subtle body, much as we today map ocean currents, air currents, and even global lines of magnetic strength. They even offer us a picture of the process by which the Infinite becomes the finite cosmos. In this chapter, we will look at these yogic maps.

The Infinite's Five Powers

One of the most beautiful and brilliant depictions of how the Divine forces construct our universe comes from Kashmir Shaivism, an old monistic faith. (Remember that even in this glorious tradition, the intellect, albeit refined and cleansed, attempts to comprehend and explain in words what is utterly transcendent. The mind tries to make it understandable, both so that it can be informed by the transcendent knowledge that arises within it and so that it can convey the experience of union with the Infinite for the benefit of others.) According to the Shaivite faith, God, the Infinite Auspicious One, possesses five abilities, of which all else in the cosmos is a manifestation. Shiva's (the Auspicious One's) power is inextricably linked to its creative power of Consciousness, or Shakti, which possesses the five powers: the ability to create everything, the ability to sustain that creation, the ability to destroy everything, the ability to conceal anything, and the ability to reveal anything, including Her and thus your Infinite nature. Kashmir Shaivism provides a great map of how we transition from the limitless Shakti/Shiva, unbounded in every aspect possible, to the contracted restricted finite form of who we are in this life.

These five forces are present every instant, and we can see them at work in our minds. Our minds reflect the action of these five forces inside the constrained area of our reality. We have all of the Infinite's powers, although in a weakened form. We build something in our minds and then hold it there as long as we desire. We then disintegrate and discard that shape, or we may conceal and tuck it away in our memory, revealing it again by bringing it back to consciousness. In this sense, the ordinary mind continuously reflects these five boundless capabilities of our divine essence, albeit in a restricted form.

Exercise of the Five Powers

Knowing yourself as a force at work with your five abilities is as simple as taking a moment now to observe your energies blossoming in the vast awareness of your mind.

You can build, sustain, disintegrate, conceal, and disclose. Take a minute to observe your mind in operation and identify each of these powers.

Close your eyes for a few seconds or stare into space while you direct your focus to the inner space, the inner sky of awareness, and see what you produce. Thoughts and pictures, memories and feelings originate, persist, dissipate, are hidden in your memory, or are uncovered by bringing them back to consciousness.

Continue to awe your abilities when you observe them in action. You are also generating the feeling of being a restricted form of force, playing in your mind's sandbox. In contrast, your fully expanded force nature observes with perfect delight and limitless bliss!

Enjoy this for as long as you want. You can return to this state of consciousness at any time and place, even if your mind is preoccupied with something else.

The power of revelation is intrinsic, and the process of Kundalini rising unveils this fundamental potential, which is quite intriguing and informative for comprehending Kundalini. Kundalini unveils what the power of concealment has concealed – our oneness with the Divine. This power is also known as Maya Shakti, or the ability to impose limitations. The Infinite has no boundaries; it is what it means to be infinite. Maya means "quantifiable," therefore, the Infinite takes on the restrictions inherent in all forms by using its force, Maya Shakti – the immeasurable becomes measurable, the Infinite becomes limited, and the One becomes many by its own decision. You've opted to accept your mind's and body's limits. It takes the strength of the Auspicious One to create the illusion of separation and limitation, and it takes the force of the Auspicious One to dispel that illusion. The mind alone will never be able to do this.

This map is yet another magnificent depiction of how the force of the Infinite takes on myriad limited forms, which it then comes to know by inhabiting them, entering them with consciousness. Shakti must first conceal its infinity from itself. The Infinite will not be able to fit inside the limit until it deliberately accepts that constraint. This isn't limited to the most well-known expressions of the Divine, such as Jesus, Buddha, or Krishna. This acceptance of restriction is true of all forms, from the electrons in the atoms that comprise this word to the entire cosmos. On an individual level, the power of concealment provides for the conscious sense of restrictions and separation, the bounds of "I am a man," "I am a woman," "I am a kid," or whatever constrained container. "I" awareness enters through identification. Our Infinite essence is unlimited "I-Consciousness." Its ability to hide helps it understand the constraints of the finite universe it generates. Your ordinary finite self, who you've always thought of yourself as, is the Divine understanding of what it's like to be you and choosing to be you as you.

As the force of grace and disclosure, Kundalini opposes the power of concealment. The complete experience of ourselves and the entire universe at one with the Divine is the objective of Kundalini's awakening. Full Kundalini Awakening is the Divine deciding to recognize Itself as both limited and infinite at the same time.

Contemplation

To further grasp this process, envision a great deep ocean that is peaceful and still as the Divine's Infinite Consciousness. God continues to create, and a wave develops on the ocean, a form that has its existence while being one with the water. Now assume that the wave's oneness with the ocean is hidden from it and that the wave is given liberty to experiment with other shapes. As a wave of Consciousness, the wave is conscious in a limited sense and perceives itself as a vast wave, then a little wave, a ripple, a tall wave, a fat wave, and so on. It is changing one's shape and taking on a new one. However, like with many pastimes, this becomes tedious after a while. The wave has learned everything through changing shapes, and it is no longer creative or significant enough to continue doing so. The wave has a vague sense of being a part of something bigger and begins to yearn for something bigger. It longs to be reunited with the sea, with God. This is where God's fifth power, the power of grace and revelation, enters the picture. Through grace, God undoes the work of its concealment power and reveals the truth of unbroken unity with God. The wave enjoys reflecting the ocean. The illusion of separation is dispelled, and it experiences the thrill of oneness with our Creator once more.

In response to this deception, the fifteenth-century poet Saint Kabir wrote:

Rising, water's still water,

falling back, it is water,

will you give me a hint how

to tell them apart?

The explanations of Shakti Kundalini's five-fold strength and how the malas shroud our infinite nature provide us the wisdom we need to see beyond the blinding intricacies of all the forms that arise in the mind and the world. Regaining our Self, Shakti Kundalini's viewpoint, we can observe the beautiful dynamics of creation unfolding, producing all these forms from the one essence, Shakti. It's like wandering into a massive jewelry store and seeing all of the gold necklaces, bracelets, rings, charms, and earrings, then taking a step back and seeing all the gold in all the display cases, gleaming in varied shapes, forms, and purposes while staying, simply, gold. Nothing exists that is not Shakti Kundalini!

Symbol of the Divine Within the Coiled Serpent

The force of Kundalini is there in everyone, but it remains dormant until the big awakening, which is the holiest event in the soul's journey back to its source. Kundalini is sometimes described symbolically in yogic scriptures as a coiled snake sleeping inside us, a serpent whose excellent capabilities manifest when it awakens and uncoils. During meditation, one may even perceive the archetypal shape of a coiled snake, which is the source of Kundalini's name. The snake, a sign of the Divine Feminine, and the lingam, a symbol of the Divine Masculine, around which the snake is entwined, are ancient symbols of the Infinite as Shakti/Shiva in the root chakra, the Muladhara. The snake and lingam represent the divine union of female and male, Holy Mother and Holy Father, as completely present throughout creation, from the endlessly expanding formless, transcendent world of the Sahasrara (crown chakra) to the terrestrial realm of bound forms in the Muladhara.

This may appear impossible, but it isn't. It's fantastic that each human has a spiral form of bound energy that contains more knowledge than the world's top scientists can fathom. When the two parts of the spiral are linked to form a whole, this spiral form of bound energy wakes and begins to disclose its incomprehensible knowledge.

This spiral form of confined energy within you is invisible to you. It is minuscule, but it can grow a fully human person from a single cell. It directed the growth of a single, infinitesimally speck of protoplasm into the trillions of distinct cells that comprise your body. This spiral form of bound energy figured out how to turn that one minuscule particle of living stuff into your heart, lungs, nerves, brain, eyes, ears, nose, skin, teeth, bones, and muscles. It then produced all types of cells, including white blood cells, red blood cells, nerve and muscle cells, bone and cartilage cells. It knew when to cease growing them and where to plant them. It allows your fingernails but not your fingers to grow; it enables your hair but not your ears to grow, and it extends your heart in the appropriate spot and connects it to your head. It understood exactly where each artery and vein should grow in your complete circulatory system. It understood just where to create the nerve cells that travel from your big toe to your brain and back again.

Is this too fantastic to be true? Do I expect you to think that a small, spiral form of bound energy can do all of this? Yes! We don't know how, but we do know that DNA, the spiral form of bound energy that makes up your genes, drives the remarkable evolution of a single cell into the unfathomably intricate structure of trillions of cells known as the human body. What makes you think a little Consciousness couldn't be lying dormant within you — symbolically represented as a coiled serpent, waiting to propel your awareness back to union with the Creator, if the universe's energy can be bound in the molecules forming DNA, subtly encode all the information necessary to create from itself the many diverse organs, tissues, and cells of the body and have them successfully operate together? DNA is not Kundalini, but it demonstrates how a large quantity of information — the structuring and functioning of every cell and the biochemistry inside billions of cells — can be packed into something so little that it appears unnoticeable to the human eye. Kundalini is within you, even if you are unaware of its presence. Maybe she's already waking up from her rest!

The Soul's Evolution Throughout Life

What is the process by which awareness evolves, and what is the soul learning across countless lives and various life-forms? In the yogic tradition, awareness grows across innumerable lives and includes incarnations in multiple life forms. The yogic practice also gives a map or depiction of how the evolutionary process develops. One way to think about this is to visualize a circle and the cyclical pattern as the soul's learning journey through many incarnations.

As you can see, the right side of the circle is in the process of involution. This "outgoing phase" (from twelve to six o'clock) is known as savritti, while the "return phase" (from six to twelve) is known as nivritti. The savritti stage of the cycle is where the soul or awareness evolves and takes on forms. It is learning what it means to be an individualized awareness. This is done by journeying through all of the innumerable incarnations and learning from each one about the consequences of its actions, the causes of pain, the power of love, the dynamics of creation, etc. It is experiencing the many things we might encounter in life, in the afterlife. The second part of the voyage, nivritti, represents the transformation that occurs due to shedding forms. This is the process of getting rid of affiliation with bound structures, cleaning away karmas while attempting to produce as little new karma as possible, and only positive karma. The nivritti phase begins with the initial Kundalini stirrings and lasts until awareness regains the totality of its actual unbounded nature in a live state of radical liberation, living samadhi. The pravritti-nivritti cycle charts the growth of the soul across many incarnations.

The soul states to itself near the conclusion of the savritti phase, "I've learned enough; I've been through the endless cycles of birth and death; I've learned so many things through that, but the pain is tiresome. The absence of actual freedom is just too restricting. The enduring fullness, unbreakable joy, and unlimited love that I want will never be obtained in this way." The soul senses that there is much more to life at this stage. There's a lot more to who we are and what we are than living within the confines of a mind and a body, identifying as a man or a woman, young or old, and all the other things we take for granted as defining who we are. We begin to understand that no matter how much we possess and consume, joy is transitory, power is transient, and old age, decline, and death are unavoidable. We begin to suspect that there was an original experience of being linked with something more profound, everlasting, blissful, and calm. How do we reclaim it?

That time of waking is the transition point in the soul's evolutionary cycle between venturing forth to study everything that happens with contracting and taking on forms and returning to the cycle when the soul goes through expanding and shedding forms. At this point in the cycle, we call upon our intrinsic ability to know the Self to reawaken. It is time for grace to descend. For the Holy Spirit to rebaptize the soul, for bodhicitta to ascend and outshine the conditioned intellect. It is time for the most auspicious event — shaktipat.

Shaktipat is frequently depicted as a lightning bolt. Just as lightning only strikes the ground when there is a charge buildup in both the earth below and the sky above, we build the charge of seeking to be free of the endless death and rebirth cycles that accompany the savritti phase in the ground of our soul.

That entire cycle of taking on forms and releasing them is not just one that unfolds throughout countless lives; it also occurs inside each existence. Look at what happens from the time we are born until we mature and pass away: Notice the vast amount of growth and change, expansion and contraction, which occurs as we try on different identities — first as an infant, then as a child, then as an adolescent, then as a student, an employee, and in relationships. We may investigate what it means to be a husband, wife, or partner, a father or mother within each life. We explore what happens to our consciousness as it fills the identity containers associated with those various roles. As we grow older and more comfortable with our roles and identities, there will inevitably come a time when we will begin to distance ourselves from them. Some fade with time. For example, we must transition from adolescence to adulthood, graduate from high school, be fired, divorced, or suffer from an accident or disease that prevents us from functioning. We are forced to let go of certain identities until, eventually, at death, we shed even the body. That same process, that same arc of development that involves taking on forms of our creation and dissolving them, occurs throughout each lifetime.

Every day, the same pattern repeats itself. When you wake up in the morning, you begin to play roles. You could start your day by asking yourself, "What do I have to do today?" and then you put on the part of your job. Maybe it's a day off, and you're thinking, "Oh, what am I going to do with my kids, or with my husband, or by myself?" We take on a different role for each relationship, a different identity, or a different aspect of our identity. We may even put on the clothing that corresponds to that role identity.

If we're heading to work, we may wear a uniform, whether a suit and tie or another type of uniform connected with that position. We adopt that role as we put it on, and our awareness enters it, and we get the experience of assuming that part. "I am _____" is the thought-form associated with this process of identification, the process of consciousness pouring itself into the containers: I am a professional, I am unemployed, I am a mother, I am a man, I am a woman, and so on. We go through the entire day in this manner, and then there comes the point later in the day when it's time to start shedding those roles, those identities. We could do it on the way home, or when we come into our bedroom, take off the uniform we wore all day, and put on something light and comfy.

When the day draws to a close, we put on our sleeping garments, another symbolic change in outfits. To transition from the usual waking state to the sleep state, we must physically shed and lose all of those roles and identities. If we cannot shed all of our everyday duties, we may be unable to fall asleep. We might be irritated, anxious, or thrilled. We might have to do something to let go of the day and everything we've taken on, shift states, and fall asleep. When we can't let go, when the conditioned mind is so connected and clinging to the objects of the day, when the brain won't disengage, we may resort to drugs to wipe away the waking state mind and erase all the enervation that comes from identifying with this or that function. We desire a release from the limitations and tensions of the forms we've taken on all day, such as the savritti phase of involution and the nivritti phase of letting go, which will bring us more peace and satisfaction.

On the other hand, ordinary sleep lacks the enlarged consciousness of awakened Kundalini; the relaxation is short. The following morning we're back on the treadmill, pursuing sparkling delights and dreams, taking on constrained identities to engage in their quest. Kundalini's awakening brings you to a condition of profound liberation that is already waiting for you, just beyond deep slumber and the dreamy life of the ordinary mind.

Awakening

The analogy of awakening from sleep is a great approach to explain what happens when Kundalini activates. Imagine you're sound asleep when your alarm goes off or your dog jumps on the bed, and you've gone from one reality — the reality of a deep slumber or a dream — to the waking state reality of lying in your bed. You realize you've awoken to what was previously completely present, the world around you, but you're now awake, conscious, and experiencing it directly. You can be in a dream reality one minute and then awaken to the everyday reality of your waking world the next, which was already fully there, but you were unaware of it throughout your deep sleep or dreams. Kundalini Awakening allows us to immediately experience the presence already there — the Divine, the Infinite presence that already exists entirely. It doesn't appear out of nowhere; we're simply and fully awakening to our undivided unity with God. Though awakening is a metaphor, it is important because it gives a picture, a map, of transitioning from a state of unconsciousness or dreams to a state of awareness in which we understand what was already fully there.

Directly recognizing our connection with every human being, our deep connection with nature, and our sense of unity with All are some of the ways that the waking experience may manifest itself. Some people experience awakening while walking in the woods and suddenly feel a profound connection to every living presence, including trees, shrubs, birds, bugs, and even the rocks. Another person may experience this sense of connection while standing in the middle of Grand Central Station; suddenly, the quality of sound, the vitality of people, and everything around them become part of their awakened experience of being at one with the flow of all of that life, all of that hustle and bustle, all of the universes that every person represents — their suffering, pains, longings, happiness, and their intimate connection with all.

We can join with that Source consciously by meditating, liberating ourselves from the typical ego thought. Kundalini Shakti, the power of Consciousness that may modify and inform the totality of our waking state lives and our dream worlds, is the intrinsic power that permits us to do so. Then we can awaken to our true Self, our true nature, and go about our daily lives. From a completely different level of consciousness, with the ego-mind informed by the fullness of our Infinite nature, imbued with boundless patience, wisdom, love, and compassion for all.

The ordinary ego-mind must be closed to the Infinitude to function in waking state reality. That is its function. A mental disorder is diagnosed when a person fails to identify boundaries and limitations in their daily functioning. The problem isn't a healthy ego-mind; it's the conditioned, habitual identification with only the ego-mind that disconnects us experientially from the boundlessness of our original Being. It drives the ego-mind to act in ignorance of the sublime nature of the world, others, and ourselves — all united in Being. The uneducated ego-mind moves from one condition of need and want to fleeting fulfillment and then to the next state of lack and want. You can only abide in peace, contentment, and ecstasy if you come to rest in the infinite fullness of your true nature. Only then will you be free, fully awake, a Buddha, a Knower, a tathagata, a person who has gone beyond.

Kundalini forms the vehicles of our mind and body. It occupies them for innumerable cycles of birth and death, studying all that can be understood about the joys and hardships of everyday life via them. Kundalini also creates the road to restoring the Unity Consciousness, which extinguishes the fires of pain and yearning in an ocean of love and bliss. The mind and body are thus moved by wisdom and genuine understanding rather than ignorance and insatiable appetites. The mind/subtle body and the physical body are both vehicles that may serve either ignorance and desires or knowledge and love. Kundalini gives you the ability to make good decisions.

Kundalini: Source of Causal, Subtle, and Physical Body

Many specifics of how the Infinite creates the finite physical world of forms, such as the human body, are mapped out in the yogic tradition. It begins with the rejection of Unity Consciousness, followed by the negation of limitless power and everlasting life via the five powers and the imposition of the three malas, or coverings. This first rejection of infinity establishes the boundaries of space and time within which creation occurs. The causal body is a constrained space and time where our Infinitude has been denied. Still, the plurality of limited forms has yet to emerge — aptly named, since it is responsible for everything that follows: the formation of infinite shapes and wants, the driving force behind creation, the yearning to find what was lost. In profound sleep, the causal body is seen as a constant awareness of emptiness. The Infinite's light has been neutralized, and no creatures have yet emerged. The darkness and emptiness of deep sleep mirror this condition of nothingness; no shapes have arisen for the mind to perceive. There is a faint germ of limited I-awareness, but there is insufficient consciousness to detect it. All the ordinary mind understands about the causal condition of deep sleep is that there is a thread of self-awareness that runs through the unconsciousness of that state. It will become apparent when one experiences this stage in meditation with Kundalini's grace.

The subtle body emerges from the causal body to serve as a vehicle for experiencing constraints, desires, actions, and the lessons that awareness will learn across infinite incarnations. The ordinary mind most thoroughly perceives the subtle body during dream sleep. Kundalini can illuminate the subtle body more thoroughly in meditation with its small light of consciousness than the regular intellect can. The subtle body creates the physical body. Each of the bodily senses and organs derives from a fundamental ingredient of the subtle body.

The chakras, or working centers of consciousness, are located within the subtle body along the Sushumna Nadi. Like the nerve centers along the spinal cord, the chakras are located along the Sushumna Nadi at intersections with minor nadis.

Chakra is a Sanskrit term that means "circle" or "wheel" and is the basis of the words *circus* and *circle* in English. During meditation, the chakras may appear to the inner eye as wheels of energy or light, and they are also characterized as lotus flowers with varying numbers of petals. The energy pathways that cross at a chakra resemble the petals of a flower. The thousand-petaled lotus of the Sahasrara is the highest center, which is technically not a chakra but is usually regarded as one. These energy centers are truly active centers of awareness since the energy in the subtle body is conscious energy. The descent of consciousness is from the Sahasrara, the transcendent domain of pure Consciousness above the Sushumna Nadi, to the energy center at the base, known as the Muladhara, the earth realm. This represents the process of consciousness moving from the highest transcendent Unity Consciousness to the limitations of embodied consciousness that you and I usually experience as we live our lives in the world.

The Muladhara chakra represents the element of earth and is the last destination of Divine Consciousness, Kundalini Shakti, as it descends and manifests the world. After generating the planet and embodied existence, Kundalini rests within this chakra. As the wave dissolves back into the sea, She awaits the Great Awakening, which will reverse this process, erasing the restrictions that consciousness has taken on and allowing us to be aware of our transcendent, limitless, divine nature.

The process of involution is the descent of consciousness from the formless transcendent Godhead to the earthly realm of human existence. As consciousness ascends through the chakras, it becomes increasingly free of limitations, restrictions, and the illusion of being bound and separate from its source — God/Goddess.

The seven major chakras are Sahasrara at the crown of the head, Ajna chakra between the eyes, Vishuddha chakra in the throat, Anahata chakra near the heart, Manipura chakra near the solar plexus, Svadhishthana chakra at the root of the sexual organs, and Muladhara chakra at the base of the pelvis. The involution of consciousness from the transcendent realm of the Sahasrara to the Muladhara is represented by the progressive order of the elements that each chakra represents. Involution is how consciousness coalesces and grows grosser, denser, and more limited.

The Ajna chakra, or "Third Eye," is located just below the Sahasrara between and above our physical eyes. This is the realm of pure individualized mind. At this phase, consciousness has shed its formless, all-encompassing universality but has not yet crystallized into the physical universe. Here, consciousness may be experienced simply as a limited sense of "I-ness" that lacks the characteristics we normally associate with ourselves, such as gender, body shape, and role.

The five chakras that follow represent the manifestation of the five elements that comprise the physical realm and increasingly contracted states of consciousness, emotional patterns, and other things. The subtle elements that make up the entire human body are housed in these subtle body centers. They aren't the actual elements themselves, but the subtle energy concept is underlying the physical reality of these components: space, air, fire, water, and earth. The subtle body is entirely made up of energies; there are no gross physical components and nothing that can be measured with physical instruments, which stymies scientific efforts to study it. Only correlations of its activity reflected in physical body changes may be assessed. Yogis, as inner-world researchers, improve their awareness via meditation and the grace of Kundalini Shakti. They were and still are capable of directly seeing and mapping the subtle body. You have the same intrinsic aptitude, albeit researching the subtle body is not essential and may be a diversion from accomplishing the aim of Kundalini emerging.

There is a development from the subtlest to the grossest of the components in declining order. Looking at the elements, the vishuddha chakra, located at the throat level, represents the element of ether or space, the subtlest of the physical components. Following this, awareness descends to the Anahata chakra, the heart chakra, and the air element, as consciousness becomes denser and grosser than it was at the level represented by space. The Manipura chakra, which means the element of fire, comes next. Fire retains its subtlety, but it has more definition and is grosser than air. Following that is the Svadhishthana chakra, which represents the element water. Water is heavier and more solid than fire but not as gross and dense as earth, the final element related to the Muladhara chakra at the base of the Sushumna Nadi. At this level, we've gotten to the densest, grossest, most limiting, and constrained form of awareness, the earthy physical realm.

As a result, everything from the most subtle feeling of Infinite I-awareness to the actual world of terrestrial matter is composed of consciousness in various states of contraction. The whole force and presence of God, Divine Consciousness, are present even within the most restricted forms of physical reality. The release of that bound energy is analogous to the release of potential energy bound in matter, which results in the unexpected power and light of nuclear reactions. Kundalini Awakening releases the Divine's bound force and light that are inside the human form.

When Kundalini awakens — that is, when our awareness expands beyond the limitations of body and mind — the energy of Consciousness, also known as Shakti, ascends the Sushumna Nadi and pierces the chakras in ascending order. However, it can reverse order and revisit chakras repeatedly, in any order, while clearing outbound patterns of energy and consciousness. Overall, Kundalini Shakti expands from the solid confines of the earth realm, shedding limitations until it reaches the unbounded realm of the Sahasrara once more. The finite is united with the infinite once again, and we are reunited with the Divine, the Self of All. The last steps occur beyond the mind, beyond language, beyond the power of mind and words to capture that experience and speak about it. The entirety of Being is known in stillness.

You'd require maps illustrating ocean depths and where mountains rise from the seafloor to form islands if you plan to navigate the Pacific Ocean. You would need to know where the dangerous reefs lay below the waves, jeopardizing your safe travel. You would require charts of sea currents and prevailing winds, and of course, you would want someone who has gone across and back to help you navigate. The maps that sages and yogis brought back from crossing the ocean of samsara, of delusion and ignorance, to help others cross safely are what we have in the depictions of the five powers.

The malas and the bodies — causal, subtle, and gross — represent the condensing and contracting of the Infinite One to form the finite manifold forms of the gross body. Awakened Kundalini permits us to recognize that fully, revel in all of it as our Self, and restore the direct experience of our ever-present, never broken, all-encompassing completeness. Maps of the chakras, nadis, and subtle body guide us on the path to fully expanded consciousness.

Decoration of the Symbols in Kundalini's Maps

There's more to the chakras and what they represent than the brief overview I provide in this book. Each is a level of awareness, and the yogic sages have investigated and documented them. Each chakra has connected specific powers and distinctive sentiments that determine how we form our reality — our relationships, worldview, sense of self, and methods of interacting with the world — while working from that level chakra. The petals of each chakra vibrate with a distinct letter of the Sanskrit alphabet, and if you add up all the petals from the Muladhara to the Ajna chakra, you obtain the fifty letters of the alphabet. Each chakra has a bija mantra, a seed mantra or syllable, and so on, layer after layer of details and symbols, all mapping out how Kundalini, the power of Consciousness, creates the microcosm of your limited mind-body self.

It is critical to remember that even the best maps do not represent the terrain. This is especially true of symbolic maps. The subtle body map is a highly symbolic map of consciousness that depicts the chakras as centers of consciousness in mandala form, root energies of elements and organs of the physical body, and the like. It's critical to understand the symbolic nature of these depictions, especially since much of what's written about Kundalini, chakras, nadis, and so on, whether in books or on websites, make this all seem very concrete as if you could visualize these descriptions and you'd have it. Why would yogis devote eons to complex sadhana practices to experience these things when direct knowledge is simply obtained?

Chakras may be shown in highly concrete shapes, such as a lotus with many petals; however, they are not physical manifestations of the power of Consciousness, Kundalini Shakti. Chakras are a diverse collection of consciousness, symbols, and subtle energies outside the physical realm. There is nothing tangible about a chakra. It's especially important to understand the difference between concrete forms and symbols.

Symbols point beyond themselves and have been employed for thousands of years in mythology, religions, shamanic traditions, and other esoteric traditions such as Masonry and Kabbalah to transfer lessons, power, and energy and shield teachings practices from the uninitiated. A symbol can represent a state of awareness, an instruction, a process, or even a route that cannot be articulated precisely in words. This can be anything as basic as a black dot — a point called the Bindu that is commonly at the heart of a yantra (a complex visual symbol used for entering specific meditations) (a complex visual symbol used for entering certain meditations). That Bindu represents the gateway through which awareness must pass to transcend even the symbolic realm and enter the boundless expanse beyond language, the mind, and what even a symbol can point to. However, if we mistake a symbol for a sign, for example, thinking, "There's a six-pointed star, that's Jewish." We lose the meaning of the downward-pointing triangle as symbolic of the Divine Feminine. The upward-pointing triangle is symbolic of the Divine Masculine. The combination symbolizes the Divine union present throughout creation (a symbol of that union you'll find in yantras and chakras). It is more than just a symbol of Jewish tradition. It has great symbolic value both inside and outside of the Jewish tradition.

When we come across all of these incredible symbols and symbolic maps of awareness as we explore the depths of Kundalini, it is critical to realize that they are highly symbolic representations of Consciousness taking on form. The Zen tradition simply says, "Don't confuse the finger for the moon." The finger points to the moon, yet it isn't the moon. Teachings, conceptions, and symbols all may point to the full light of Consciousness, but they aren't it. A sign points to something outside itself; it's not that thing. Simply comprehending the instruction, the notion, or the symbol doesn't give one the moon.

This type of symbolic thinking is also necessary for comprehending these maps. Sages and seers express themselves metaphorically as a means of safeguarding their teachings. Because the power and truth of the teachings are embedded in symbols that an inexperienced person cannot comprehend, the symbolically encoded teachings are referred to as self-protecting. All their concrete thinking about it, no matter how many years or lifetimes they devote to it, will never reveal the sign's power. It's one of the reasons why it's always been vital to learn with someone who knows the teachings, fully experiences them, and can pass on everything that lies beyond the symbol, beyond what one could discover in a book or text, or on the Internet. As a result, many traditions have codified the process of transmitting the power required to accept the teachings completely. In Tibetan Buddhism, empowerments are given ritually and symbolically before the teachings, precisely because the teachings would not be comprehended and potent without empowerment.

Typically, our regular mind views things with the ego's arrogance. The ego will pursue its desires regardless of the consequences. It does not even consider a humble and respectful approach or a devotional approach. The best way to receive Kundalini's great gifts is to approach Her with reverence and humbly accept all of her gifts — whatever they may be. It requires trust and faith. That lesson is typically one that the ego-mind has a tough time with regardless of whether it is approaching Kundalini for the first time or has already been on Kundalini's road for years. Love is the best approach to becoming close to someone. Approach the Divine inside you with love, treasure her gifts with love, and merge in Her with love.

CHAPTER 4: WESTERN PSYCHOLOGY
& YOGA PSYCHOLOGY

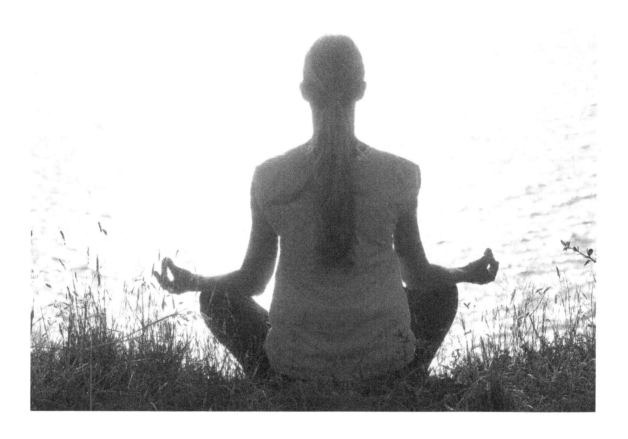

The ancient psychology of yoga provides numerous insights into how the mind and awareness function — many of which are opposed to Western psychology's paradigm on how the mind and consciousness function. Our culture is so ingrained in psychology that most individuals are unaware of it. For example, suppose someone behaved badly or oddly during another period or in another culture. In that case, their behavior might have been explained by influences from the stars or planets or blamed on demons or possessions. In other societies, it would have been ascribed to spells and witchcraft. If someone acts weirdly or abnormally in our society, we hypothesize about unpleasant childhood experiences, upbringing, familial influences, or what they've been rewarded for and learned from peer groups. We can even ask if a brain ailment or tumor causes such behavior. Our explanations are both physiological and psychological. They are immensely helpful in their own right, so they are the prevailing paradigm. We function under a Western psychological framework, oblivious to its ramifications. As a result, it's critical to examine some of the fundamental assumptions of orthodox Western psychology.

These are assumptions that many of us have without being aware of them or having recently deliberately evaluated them. It is a set of beliefs and ideas about how our minds and awareness work that may conflict with those of yoga and other Eastern and Western spiritual traditions. Misperceptions and misunderstandings can occur when multiple paradigms collide, such as our unconscious Western psychological one and a spiritual or yogic one. Understanding one's paradigm and the assumptions of the opposing paradigm might assist in preventing misperceptions and miscommunications between the two.

The physicist, historian, and philosopher of science Thomas Samuel Kuhn notably wrote about paradigm conflicts in the history of scientific evolution. A paradigm is a set of ideas, conceptions, values, and inquiry procedures that dominate the thinking of a culture — scientific, yogic, religious, or otherwise — during a specific moment in its history. Over time, the prevailing paradigm's essential assumptions become implicit and automatically arrange one's thinking, perception, and ideas about the nature of reality. For example, who considers gravity to be a potentially incorrect theory? Because of the efficacy of the theoretical conceptions of gravity, they are assumed to be "actual" and not merely theory. We still don't know what causes the mass to gravitate or where the force of gravity originates.

Kuhn argued that bringing together two divergent paradigms for comparative study or integration frequently resulted in "paradigm collision" in the history of science. When evaluating the opposing paradigm, the prevailing paradigm's implicit, unacknowledged core assumptions lead to inaccurate inferences and conclusions. On the one hand, Eastern, yogic, and transpersonal perspectives and standard Western psychological paradigms are in such a state of conflict. Unless the fundamental assumptions of each system are understood and considered during any comparisons, paradigm clash and the resulting distortions or incorrect judgments occur.

Traditional Western psychology is primarily concerned with psychology's cognitive-behavioral and psychoanalytic schools of thought. In contrast to those systems of thinking, Yoga psychology varies the most. Humanistic and transpersonal psychology are two more significant schools of psychology. On the level of fundamental assumptions, yoga psychology is more akin to them and indistinguishable from transpersonal psychology. Yoga psychology refers to the system defined by Patanjali (the great sage and codifier of yoga around two thousand years ago) and implemented via the non-dualistic systems of Advaita Vedanta and Kashmir Shaivism.

When comparing a more significant, more inclusive paradigm to a smaller, more restricted one, we get misconceptions and incorrect conclusions. In its view of the range of functioning of human consciousness, the multiple states of consciousness model held by meditation disciplines or consciousness disciplines, including yoga and other traditions of meditation or prayer, are significantly broader than the traditional Western psychological one. When the Western paradigm is applied to Kundalini, yoga, or the consciousness disciplines, these Eastern psycho-spiritual systems and the aspects of consciousness they describe may be perceived as unhealthy or illogical and simply branded or discarded as unreal.

Traditional Western psychology is similar to the consciousness disciplines in the same way Newtonian physics is to Einsteinian physics: It is a subset of the larger, more encompassing paradigm. Transpersonal psychology is a paradigm that seeks to incorporate and integrate the full spectrum of human functioning, from the most sublime states studied by consciousness sciences to the most confined pathological conditions described by standard Western psychology.

Four essential issues emphasize the fundamental distinctions between the paradigms of yogic or awareness sciences and standard Western psychology:

1. Whether our typical, awake state of awareness is optimum or suboptimal
2. The existence of actual higher levels of awareness
3. Whether or if training may lead to higher levels of awareness
4. Whether or whether verbal communication is sufficient for communicating information, particularly knowledge obtained from higher levels of awareness

The consciousness sciences believe that the waking state is suboptimal, that higher states of consciousness exist and may be achieved and that linguistic communication about them is restricted. According to traditional Western psychology, the waking state is the best state of consciousness; other states are suboptimal, irrelevant, or diseased, and intellectual analysis based on the verbal encoding of experience is the greatest form of knowledge.

Before the advent of quantum physics, traditional Western psychology reflected the materialistic philosophical perspective characteristic of the physical sciences. The materialist viewpoint is most visible in Freudian and cognitive-behavioral psychology. Both seek the material, the physiological, to explain human nature. Even Freud, who brought to light the unconscious mind's enormous influence on the conscious mind, was a materialist, noting, "All our provisional concepts in psychology will someday be grounded on a biological substrate." Many psychiatrists, neurologists, neuropsychologists, and psychologists feel we've arrived at that stage. They believe they can write about Buddha's brain and explain his consciousness based on brain function, thereby denying the possibility of past incarnations or the growth of consciousness through life. Materialist science holds that our physical body and brain are the only things that determine us. A materialist scientist would constantly try to reduce consciousness and Kundalini to physical occurrences and processes. Many people believe that Photon emissions and other physical processes create Kundalini. This just reflects material science's limits and the reductionism of scientific researchers. According to the yogic and contemplative practices, consciousness resides outside the material brain. This is a key issue of contention.

Traditional Western psychology attempts to explain the subtle in terms of the gross, claiming that the gross, physical level of reality (physiology, brain chemistry, sensory functioning, and so on) produces the subtler phenomenon of consciousness (awareness, consciousness, intuitions, etc.). As a result, under such psychologies, the spectrum of authentic human experience is confined to those associated with material existence. Traditional Western psychology dismisses altered states of consciousness, mystical states of unity and ecstasy, trans-body or out-of-body experiences, post-death experiences, and transpersonal experiences as pathological, regressive, or purely subjective. At times, behaviorists have neglected or rejected the presence of consciousness, dismissing it as a simple side effect of bodily functioning. Yoga psychology has significantly impacted the newer Western psychologies, humanistic and transpersonal, incorporating Eastern psychological notions into their frameworks.

Basic Assumptions in Yoga vs. Western Psychology

Yoga's ideas about the body differ from those of Western psychology.

1. The universe's nature
2. Consciousness's nature
3. The human being's nature
4. The levels at which the human mind functions
5. The underlying causes of human sorrow
6. How one obtains respite from pain

You might find it fascinating to pause and consider your thoughts and opinions about these six topics.

According to yoga, there is only one "stuff" in the cosmos: pure unbounded Consciousness, also known as the Infinite Spirit of God, or Shakti. As a result, it is monistic rather than just monotheistic. In the yogic tradition, pure implies free of any limiting form of duality, which means there are no pairs of opposites, no subject-object divide, no self and other; all that exists is the Self of All — God, Shiva, Shakti, the One. Yoga claims that pure Consciousness shrinks to become the cosmos, similar to how physicists believe energy takes the shape of matter. Consciousness is the nature of the cosmos; every wave, every atom is an expression of Consciousness. Thus, the subtle generates the gross, and consciousness creates the body and exists irrespective of it.

Yoga psychology considers healthy human functioning to include a wide range of states of consciousness and experiences that go beyond physical awareness. Like many spiritual disciplines, it specifies precise strategies for experiencing who we are beyond our body and intellect. According to orthodox Western psychology, awareness cannot exist independently of the body because consciousness is thought to be physically created and physiologically based.

Yoga teaches us that:

1. The universe's essence is pure Consciousness manifested in various forms or levels of contraction.
2. Though beyond words, the nature of pure Consciousness is defined as endless, infinite Being, Consciousness, and Bliss. Consciousness reflects the features of a limiting form when it identifies with it — whether it is inanimate, vegetative, animal, human, or transcendent.
3. A human being's fundamental essence is pure Consciousness, the nameless Infinite that wears countless names.
4. The mind operates on several levels, defined by the three stages of consciousness recognized by Western psychology (waking, dreaming, and profound sleep). A fourth, acknowledged by yoga, is the infinite state of the Self, known as the turiya state.

5. There are two causes of human suffering: the relative cause and the absolute cause. The relative cause is a lack of fundamental necessities such as food, shelter, and warmth. This is also a belief held by Western psychology. The absolute source of suffering is ignorance of the Self, incorrect identification, and thinking of ourselves as the mind-body complex rather than the Self of All, the Infinite, or Buddha mind.

6. Yoga focuses on the source of all pain, which can only be alleviated by directly understanding our actual identity with the Divine. Yoga, in its entirety, seeks to bring about the understanding and experience of our genuine basic essence as pure limitless Consciousness.

Working toward Self-realization is, indeed, regarded as the ultimate human activity and the particular goal of all yoga practices. According to yoga psychology, we are as much rooted in the richness and completeness of our ultimate Self as we are in the limiting and desiring character of our bound Self. This is in stark contrast to Freud's idea of effective psychotherapy as "transforming the neurotic's severe suffering into the usual sorrow of human existence." Western psychology is still in the early phases of creating cognitive-behavioral approaches to positive psychology and health psychology, yet its fundamental assumptions remain materialist.

Yoga psychology accepts three typical states of consciousness and a fourth, the turiya state of super-consciousness or Self-awareness. Its waking state is significantly constrained, if not a condition of illusion, than the turiya state. Turiya is the Self's ever-present, pure I-consciousness, the witness of the three normal states of consciousness. It is the highest level of Consciousness, described by mystics of all religions as a euphoric state of complete oneness. Turiya is the state that encompasses the other three states and illuminates them with Consciousness. Adepts see Turiya awareness as everlasting, uncaused, omniscient, and ubiquitous. It cannot be distinguished from the Self. The true essence of the turiya condition is incomprehensible, impenetrable by speech, words, or the ordinary intellect.

Typically, we only encounter a tiny portion of turiya in the shape of a continuous sensation of I-ness that endures despite the discontinuity of the numerous states of thought and awareness that comprise reality. We may suspect that there is more to ourselves than we realize, but the ultimate immensity, the boundless breadth of our I-ness, our Selfhood, is beyond our grasp. Trying to know the Self with the intellect is akin to attempting to illuminate the sun with a shattered piece of a mirror. The basic characteristic of Consciousness in the Self allows the Self to be the illuminating source behind the intellect, senses, and body. Knowing the pure "I" in its entirety, according to yogic psychology, is the most significant objective and purpose of human growth.

The ultimate level and direct experience knowledge of turiya, according to Eastern studies and yoga psychology, in particular, are beyond the mind and speech. To reach there, one must abandon the mind and logic. This argument runs counter to conventional Western psychology's core assumptions, which see thinking as the finest talent and the written word as the least ambiguous, most accurate manner of imparting our greatest knowledge. When challenged to express oneness with the Absolute, mystics of all traditions either fall quiet or turn to poetry and symbols that point beyond themselves.

Yogis have researched the many states of consciousness available to humans for thousands of years and decided that our normal waking state is one of illusion, comparable to the dream state. They arrive at this conclusion from what yoga psychology regards as the greatest state of awareness, the previously discussed turiya state. The other three states of consciousness, according to this viewpoint, are self-imposed restrictions and the antithesis of Infinite Consciousness.

Three States of Consciousness

Yoga psychology describes in several ways how the process of restricting pure transcendent Consciousness culminates in the confined state of consciousness we are familiar with. One map depicts three stages of this procedure. These three stages correlate to the three normal states of consciousness: deep sleep, dreaming, and waking up.

The deep sleep state is the causal body's state; it is the consciousness of nothingness. It is caused by the Self's power of concealment, Maya Shakti, negating the genuine, all-encompassing state of Consciousness. As previously stated, this self-negation is known as avidya (primal ignorance). It marks the start of the concept of limited individuality, the ego-sense, and connection with constraints. As a result, one considers oneself a restricted individual rather than universal and boundless. It is a denial of one's genuine nature, a denial of one's true Self, and identification with a small component of that Self. It is referred to as the causal body because the denial of, or dis-identification from, one's actual nature causes all that follows. This is the primary cause of Consciousness' contraction into the restricted forms of thought and body that we know. They develop from the fundamental denial of universality. It is the source of all pain.

There is simply the awareness of emptiness in the profound sleep stage. The Universal Self has been denied or dis-identified, so we are unaware of it. Yet, the universe of particulars and the thoughts, desires, and specifics of human existence have not arisen. This condition, lit by Kundalini Shakti, may be distinctly experienced in meditation. We experience it in deep sleep, but since we are detached from our fully conscious, observing Self, our perception of it is simply the black vacuum of deep sleep. We know we had a profound sleep and were conscious of nothingness for a while, but we never pause to consider how that might be.

This is a famous Vedantic argument proving the presence of the Self as the conscious witness to the various states of the mind. How can we be conscious that we are aware of nothingness? What portion of us stays cognizant even when unconscious of the world, body, or mind? Who is cognizant when we dream and recount the dream to ourselves? From a yogic perspective, our Self is the ever-present, ever-conscious witness, and we can never be fully detached from it, any more than a wave can be split from the ocean. Our anguish and search stem solely from the ignorance of our oneness with it. Even when you are deep asleep, you can access yourself. The awareness of the Self, which is always present and enlightening, permits us to experience the emptiness of profound sleep and the contents of the other states of consciousness. We can re-experience our union if we transfer our focus to the Witness, the Experiencer of that condition.

The causal body gives rise to the subtle and physical bodies and their associated states of dreaming and waking. The mind, ideas, emotions, attitudes, and so on are all part of the subtle body experience. It's the subtle "I" compared to the gross "I" linked with the physical body. The dream state represents our identification with the mind and the delicate sensations that make it up. Because the subtle body is not limited by the physical rules that control the physical body, the subtle body's experiences and activities during dreams appear incomprehensible to the mind connected with the physical body in the waking state. However, while in the subtle body, one might have "paranormal," out-of-body, or post-death experiences. Such experiences may occur throughout yogic practices, particularly in meditation through activated Kundalini, and are interpreted to reflect the extension of one's consciousness beyond the boundaries of one's physical body.

Yoga psychology goes into great length on the mind and how it works. It is analogous to the many accounts of the mind and personality provided by Western psychology in several aspects. Yoga psychology, for example, incorporates ideas such as the ego, the unconscious, and processes such as projection, identification, and conditioning. However, the origin and context are quite different. The mind's relationship to bondage and liberation, its existence across time, and the condition of the mind in various stages of awareness are three of the most prominent elements of the framework in which it is seen in yoga.

Yoga considers the mind to be the source of both bondage and release. It causes bondage by believing that it is not the Self, but this specific, finite human. Individual awareness is related to Universal Consciousness. That rejection of limitless fullness generates a desiring and imperfect identity. According to yoga, the mind then produces the senses, the body, and the physical universe to explore in pursuit of fullness, completeness, and absolute identity. The Self, the almighty, appears feeble and wants power by pumping iron or climbing the corporate ladder. The omniscient seems unaware and intends to enhance its consciousness through counseling, development groups, Eastern disciplines, and courses. That which is everlasting is time-bound and attempts to evade death while leaving a legacy to be remembered.

How often have you felt like a victim of your impulses, knowing you shouldn't do something yet feel compelled to do it anyway? The unconscious is a component of the subtle body. Depth psychologists like Freud and Jung Yoga see the unconscious as a reservoir of previous experiences and the driving force behind much of an individual's current behaviors and ideas. The subtle body exists independently of the physical body and does not die like the physical body. It contains the karmic impressions, desires, and dispositions formed across many lives, not just one, as Western psychology believes.

These impressions, known as samskaras, are stored in the subtle body and govern a large portion of what we do, want, and experience in this life. The mind produces the physical body to experience the consequences of previous acts (karma) and fulfill current goals in the material world. Those ideas about the nature of the mind and its continuity from one life to the next are in direct conflict with the following basic assumptions of traditional Western psychology:

1. The physical body is the only body we have.
2. Death is the unavoidable end of human existence.
3. Physical death is the final termination of human consciousness.

In terms of how the contents of the unconscious reach there, the yogic conception varies from Freud's. Sigmund Freud believed that repression is how most unconscious information is formed. Still, yoga psychology believes that virtually every thought, desire, behavior, or experience leaves a trace regardless of whether or not it is repressed. These traces (samskaras) accumulate throughout time and serve as templates or potentialities for forming future thoughts, desires, acts, and bodies.

Yoga psychology provides an efficient approach to resolving mental issues. Given that initial impressions have accumulated throughout several lives, it is hard to identify the antecedent reasons influencing our current psychological makeup. It's pointless to go into our history and analyze tragedies indefinitely. Such a search would be futile in calming the mind and stopping those perceptions from continuing to impact it. Because the fundamental problem is core ignorance of who we are and the following modifications of the mind — the thoughts, feelings, and misguided conceptions of who we are — the remedy is to quiet the changes of the mind and eradicate the root ignorance.

All yoga techniques attempt to calm the mind and eliminate the source of ignorance. Yoga investigates and categorizes the contents of the mind and provides cures, or yogic practices, for diminishing and eliminating thought waves or mind alterations to enable one to remain in one's real nature.

All mental alterations, known as vrittis, can be grouped into one of five categories and defined as either painful or non-painful. The five sorts are as follows: correct information, incorrect knowledge, fantasy, profound sleep, and memory. In the context of yoga, the terms painful and non-painful have different connotations. Thought waves that express or perpetuate the belief that we are not the Self are painful vrittis. Thus, even your favorite chocolate cake or anything else you enjoy is regarded as unpleasant. They reinforce concepts like "I am the body, the source of my joy is external, my identity is constrained somehow, love comes from this or that." Such vrittis create wants, prompting us to seek out some items while avoiding others, keeping us trapped in the cycle of life and death. Non-painful vrittis are neutral, such as merely viewing the sky while walking, or they lead to freedom and connection with our actual Self, such as thoughts like, "I am not bound to the body, I am not restricted to the mind, I am the Self."

It's worth noting that the two major categories are "painful" and "non-painful," rather than "painful" and "pleasurable" or "joyful." This is a critical point. It expresses the yogic understanding that mental changes do not bring real pleasure, joy, or love. Ananda, or the characteristics of pleasure and love, are limitless levels of the Self.

According to yoga, when we separate ourselves from our intrinsic Ananda, our ecstasy, and our Self, we project it onto objects and others and seek it externally. We believe that eating rich, creamy, chocolate-chip ice cream will bring us delight, but the yearning for it causes our thoughts to get disturbed. When we finally stroll to the store, get home, and dig in, there's a time when the craving fades, the mind quiets, and we're lost in the ecstasy of chocolate chips! That's an example of how we may have experienced a mirror of the time when our mind was silent — devoid of ideas and wants — and we're in the joy of our Self (Ananda).

According to the yogic viewpoint, pleasure and love always originate from within. If pleasure were indeed in the chocolate ice cream, we would feel it every time we ate it, no matter how much we ate. But that's not true. We delude ourselves into thinking that pleasure, love, and joy are external qualities, rather than seeing them as emanating from within and turning our attention toward the Self. We should immerse ourselves in our innate center of love, allowing it to flow outward as naturally as a rose shares its beauty and fragrance with all passersby.

Nature of the Mind in Deluxe

The mechanism we get fooled by is simply a conditioning process comparable to those outlined in current cognitive-behavioral psychology. The sequence in the conditioning process is as follows:

1. Avidya, the primal ignorance manifested as identification with the limited self rather than the true Self, causes mental agitation of desire, obscures our true nature and the experience of all-encompassing wholeness and bliss inherent to it.
2. The desires are focused on a specific object.
3. Possession of the object temporarily eliminates the agitation caused by the desires, allowing the mind to be relative; This sensation is temporally associated with the thing, and we mistakenly assume that the object caused the delight or pleasure.

Because we are connected with our subtle and physical bodies, we are more vulnerable to indoctrination. Our attention is drawn to sensory and mental-emotional events and their interactions. Conditioning does not influence the causal body or the Self. Conditioning cannot occur in the separate stages of profound sleep and turiya. We are not conscious of any physical or mental occurrences during deep sleep, and we are beyond them during turiya. Yoga techniques may be considered deconditioning activities that dissolve the conditioning patterns created during lifetimes of identification with our brains and bodies.

All mental changes must be overcome by intensive practice and discrimination-based detachment. Discrimination in yoga refers to distinguishing between the Self and the mind, between one's actual nature and assumed, restricted nature, between the Infinite and the finite. With such skill, one may detach from the mind's and body's cravings and conditioned identities. The severe practice refers to the eight types of yogic practices known as the eight limbs — yamas, niyamas, asana, Pranayama, pratyahara, Dharana, dhyana, and samadhi. They attempt to reduce and eliminate all current mental alterations and samskaras from the past. These techniques and the yogic process cleanse the subtle body of all the impressions of previous lives, finally destroying avidya, the core ignorance of one's basic nature. They do not help or modify the Self because it is not bound and cannot be released. The intellect, on the other hand, is restricted. According to Vedanta, the mind is like a filthy mirror, with its ability to reflect reality blurred and distorted. Yogic techniques cleanse the mind of filth or vrittis, and the cleansed mind reflects the brilliant Consciousness of the Self.

According to yoga psychology, the mind assumes whatever it lingers on, just as water takes the shape of whatever container it is poured into. Our minds usually focus on the subtle and physical bodies, taking on their shapes and associating with them. As a result, consciousness is typically restricted to the body and mind and the roles and duties they perform. The mind is taken away from the physical body during meditation and directed toward the pure unbounded Consciousness of the Self. The mind that dwells on the formless Self loses its finite character and merges with Consciousness. Patanjali, all vrittis cease, and one abides in one's actual essence.

Immersion in samadhi regularly cleanses one of all samskaras, all prior perceptions of limits, and transforms one's identity from the mind-body complex to pure Consciousness. When we identify with our thoughts, we consider our limited selves to be the subject, the knower, and the perceiver of objects. Yoga teaches that the body, mind, and its contents and the states of waking, dreaming, and profound sleep are all objects of perception for a conscious knower. The Self is that aware knower who is never an object of knowledge. Never seen, it is always the Seer. Even in the middle of all the ideas and behaviors of the conventional self, the ego-mind, one's identity stays fixed in one's Self.

Dharana Mountain

Regularly doing this meditation practice can help you strengthen your ability for calm awareness and unwavering rootedness.

Begin by assuming your best meditation position, comfortable and relaxed, allowing for complete and effortless breathing. Simply follow your breath, allowing your attention to be drawn to it. As you just observe the movement of the breath and the movement of the thought, your awareness will begin to detach and step back, enabling the body to calm down. Your focus is on the inside. The mind starts to rest as your breath settles. Allow it to float on the breath's waves for a time.

Turn your focus to the feeling of heaviness in your body as it relaxes. Every breath is an invitation to the body and mind to let go, let go, let go. Your consciousness is simply watching, unattached and at peace, expansive and liberated.

Letting go and letting go makes room for now to imagine a gorgeous mountain. It may be a mountain you've seen or are familiar with, a mountain you've only seen in a picture, or a mountain that only exists in your thoughts. It is a majestic mountain that is both sturdy and stable. And it's as if you can feel the force, the solidity, the rootedness of that mountain that reaches down into the earth, to its unshakeable core, while you watch it. At the same time, as the mountain rises to new heights, it stands firm, magnificent in its magnificence.

Assume you're sitting on that mountain, comfortably perched on the ledge, experiencing the stability underneath you. Allow your consciousness to sink into that mountain, that stability sensation, and that mountain's immovable character. Unmoved, unmoved, unmoved, unmoved, unmoved, unmoved, unmoved, unmoving. Winds may blow, storms may pass, yet that mountain stands firm in its grandeur, its majesty undisturbed and unbreakable. And you profoundly inhale the solidity, majesty, and grandeur of your mountain nature.

You may sense that deep rootedness in every cell of your body, a rootedness that also sustains life, just as a vast mountain may have communities and the lives of innumerable species that rely on it. However, its unwavering, consistent excellence remains. Allow that stability, awareness, and sensation to seep into your body, all the way down into your bones, so that every cell in your body feels supported and reinforced by that unshakeable steadiness. You're entrenched in your majestic, vast nature as a magnificent creature. Inhale it thoroughly and deeply, feel its brightness infiltrate your body, providing it with power, solidity, and unwavering confidence. You can confront anything because you stay true to who you are, your exquisite Self. You're grounded in your genuine self. You may return to that sense of unshakeable rootedness as often as you like, resting there as long as you desire. Take refuge in that knowledge, an awareness that mirrors the truth of your unwavering and authentic existence.

CHAPTER 5: KUNDALINI AND MEDITATION

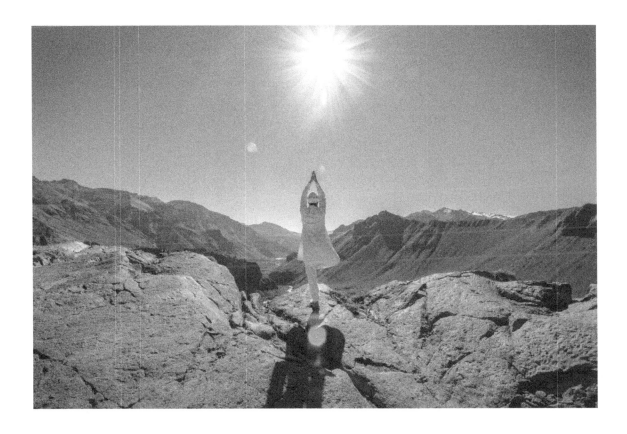

An active and deliberate technique for triggering Kundalini's awakening is meditation. To effectively use Kundalini meditation, it is necessary to grasp what meditation is.

Meditation is neither a religion nor a belief. Meditation is just a practice used by a person, regardless of religious affiliation, to develop a communication channel between himself, his body, his soul, and intellect.

Meditation helps you calm your thoughts to focus on yourself and the current moment. When you meditate, you connect with your breath and the Prana (life energy) that flows through you. Meditation creates a state of quiet that allows you to hear the callings of your soul and the cosmos. Kundalini Yoga meditation precisely supports the mind and directs the body via breathing techniques, mantra, and focus.

When you meditate, you direct your attention inside. You retain an intense concentration on and connected to your breath and vital energy. You may cleanse and purify your body, mind, and spirit by doing so. Purification is a necessary step in the Kundalini Awakening process. Purification and cleansing allow you to focus your energies, maintain a healthy body and neurological system, and keep a prayerful and loving, caring attitude.

Meditation urges you to focus on the present moment, allowing you to cleanse your subconscious, let go of the past, and entrust the future to the unknown.

Meditation allows you to become still within yourself. When you are in this profound and total level of serenity, you can recognize the ebb and flow of your thoughts and feelings without judgment or attachment. It enables you to follow your life force and energy flow freely. Kundalini is vital life energy within you. One of the many benefits of meditation for your body is to meditate on it and slowly allow it to uncoil and rise. Allowing the energy to flow freely sends it naturally and securely upwards into your crown chakra, where it will penetrate and raise you to the state of Yoga, or oneness with the Divine.

Before attempting to employ meditation to awaken your Kundalini energy, it is critical that you first get acquainted with the two essential components of this practice: the use of sounds or mantras and the use of breath or Pranayama.

Mantras

Most meditations use sounds or mantras to communicate your intentions and thoughts to the universe and yourself (from basic noises to words and phrases).

Repeatedly chanting and reciting a sound, phrase, or sentence may significantly impact the flow of ideas, feelings, and energy within you. Repeating your mantra will allow it to infiltrate your mind and body, redirecting the flow of your thoughts, emotions, and energy to where you want them to go. It enables you to absorb new beliefs and knowledge. It can reprogram how you think, feel, and use your life energy. Others may not understand what you're saying. These rules may not even be grammatically valid, yet they do not apply here. What matters is that the words and sounds you choose as your mantra will provide you with a glimpse and feel of what it's like to be in the condition you're attempting to accomplish. As a result, if you wish to let go of things holding you back and surrender to the Higher Being, you might utilize the term "let go" as your mantra. Chanting your mantra creates an energy that changes and reprograms how your mind thinks, your heart feels, and even the hormones and chemicals your body produces.

One of the most important mantras used in Kundalini Yoga is "Sat Nam." Sat is the word for truth, while Nam is the word for identity. They signify "Truth is my destiny" when combined. Chanting this mantra, according to practitioners, helps awaken and invigorate the soul. Awakening the soul activates the Kundalini energy, which is latent at the base of your spine.

Remember that "Sat Nam" is only one example of a mantra you might utilize. You are allowed to make up your motto. Don't be concerned about what the chant means to others. What is important is what it means to you. If the mantra allows you to taste and experience what it's like to be in the condition you desire, it's the one for you. Find a mantra in which you believe. Your belief in your mantra will only increase its strength and energy to arouse your Kundalini and alter your life for the better.

Pranayam

In meditation, the breath is also used to connect the ego and the current moment. Paying attention to and being aware of your breathing will help you discover concentration. When there is too much noise, turmoil, and distraction, it may be challenging to focus your attention and awareness on what you desire. Using your breath as a guide can help you find your way out of the chaos and back into a state of peace, quiet, and stillness.

Your breath is linked to your life force - the energy that flows throughout you. Being able to direct your breath to various places of your body gently will also help you to lead your life force upward until it reaches and penetrates your crown chakra, where you merge with the Divine.

Simple Methods for Learning Kriya Meditation Techniques

Have you ever wondered if it's possible to live a life of pure and permanent happiness? Can you share the Divinity's wisdom and joy while spending your life on Earth?

Kriya Yoga teachings can assist you in achieving all of these goals. Kriya Yoga is a spiritual science and practice that entails activities devised and designed to liberate the body, mind, and soul from any type of bondage and repression. Once free of impediments, a person can begin to acquire pure consciousness. Self-awareness and realization will lead to recognition of the Divinity within ourselves.

Kriya Yoga incorporates various techniques ranging from mantras to Pranayama, geared towards controlling, channeling, and diverting the life force (Prana). When the life force is correctly directed, it may provide immense tranquility, peace, and control to the body, mind, and soul.

Kriya Yoga meditation uses four fundamental practices that are proven to help awaken the spirit and Kundalini.

Concentration, Life Force, and Breath

This method focuses on preparing for meditation using breath, life force, energy, and attention. A practitioner can use this technique to draw energy into the body, then to cleanse and strengthen it. It also enables the practitioner to cleanse his thoughts and ease stress and anxiety. Going through these energization exercises is critical to achieving a state of stillness that would allow the practitioner to attain awareness. It is necessary to be calm and silent to hear the callings of the universe, and one's real Self because it is only in the calm that a person may attune his soul and energies to that who (and which) is Divine.

Kriya Yoga Method

Kriya Yoga teaches its practitioners how to manage their life force or energy (Prana) via the use of the breath (Pranayama). The spine and brain, according to practitioners, represent the tree of life. The energy runs through this tree via the chakras located on the spine. Moving, diverting, and deliberately guiding the flow of these energies up and down the spine can aid in accelerating the process of Kundalini Awakening and Divine oneness.

Concentration on Latent Powers

On the other hand, the Hong-Sau Concentration Technique can awaken latent concentration skills. When practiced daily, a person can filter out any outside noise and distractions to focus on whatever goal he is attempting to attain. As a result, if someone seeks oneness with the Divine, he can detach from all that is unrelated to his purpose. He will be able to focus his attention and energy on raising his Kundalini energy to the crown chakra.

Concentration and the Search for the True Self

The Aum Meditation Technique can assist the practitioner in using his concentration capacity to feel the Divine's all-encompassing presence. This approach expands a person's consciousness beyond the boundaries of the body, mind, and soul, allowing it to transcend all physical and human limitations and propel it into a state of self-realization and Divinity.

What Exactly is Meditation?

Regular meditation practice is essential for spiritual existence and a Kundalini Awakening. But what exactly is meditation? People frequently imagine monks who spend hours with their eyes closed and bodies unmoving, repeating mantras and feeling bizarre experiences. Some even believe it is a type of devilish behavior. So, just what is meditation? To put it simply, meditation trains and quiets the mind, releases tension, and improves attention, concentration, and prayer.

As you can see, meditation has several meanings. This is because how you perceive meditation determines its true purpose. You are not properly practicing meditation if you only see it as a stress-relieving technique. It is also important to note that meditation can be used to activate the Kundalini, improve psychic abilities, and achieve enlightenment. It is now up to you to determine how much meditation you want to incorporate into your daily life.

It is also important to note that meditation is not a demonic practice. Meditation is practiced in many religions and spiritual disciplines. It has no affiliation with any group or religion. Simply put, meditation is a discipline that anyone can practice.

It is difficult, if not impossible, to grasp meditation without first experiencing it. The only way to utterly understand what meditation is all about is to practice it daily. Let us now proceed to the next phase.

Important Guidelines

Before you begin the meditation, you need to be aware of several essential guidelines for meditating successfully. Let us go over them one by one.

Correct Posture

It is critical to maintain proper posture while meditating. There are several methods for meditating available today. Meditation can be done while lying, sitting, standing, or even walking. Every stance, however, has advantages and disadvantages. You can relax more quickly when you meditate while lying down. However, a significant issue with this position is that it is easy to fall asleep, which is an issue for many novices. Although standing and walking meditation will keep you from falling asleep, it will make it more difficult to focus since you will have to invest some physical effort to maintain these positions. Not to mention that you might get tired after a while. The sitting position is the most recommended posture for meditation. This position has the advantage of keeping you awake and concentrated while also preventing you from falling asleep. Many spiritual gurus prescribe this as the best posture. Even the great Buddha attained enlightenment while sitting in meditation. Meditation may be done while sitting in a chair or even on the floor. If you are meditating on the floor or in bed, you may want to place a pillow beneath your tailbone to make yourself more comfortable.

Maintain a Straight Spine

Whatever meditation position you choose, keep your spine straight at all times. This is critical when meditating. It allows free passage of energy through the seven major chakras. Keep in mind that your primary chakras are placed along your spinal cord. By maintaining it straight, the energy flows easily and effortlessly, which aids in raising the Kundalini. Slouching while meditating is a common error, so make sure you've taught yourself the appropriate posture before meditating. It may be tough at first to refrain from slouching, especially when sitting, but don't be disheartened. With enough practice, your body will learn to adjust, and you will become proficient. Simply keep practicing.

Focus

When you meditate, you will be asked to focus your attention on something. It might be as basic as a visualization exercise or as complex as a sound or item. Don't let your thoughts stray. Stay focused at your center of attention in a particular meditation session. If other ideas enter your head, try your best to ignore them.

A typical problem people face while learning to meditate is the monkey mind. What exactly is the monkey mind? It is a state of mind that is filled with ideas. The mind leaps from one concept to the next, just like a monkey does from one branch to another. This will undoubtedly be a struggle for those just starting to meditate. So, how do you manage the monkey mind? Keep practicing meditation. The more you meditate, the better you will be at controlling your thoughts. There are no shortcuts other than consistent practice.

Relax

While meditating, you should be as calm as possible. Allow your body to sleep and your mind to unwind. Don't think of what you're doing as difficult. This will put you under unnecessary strain and pressure, preventing you from reaching a higher level of consciousness. Simply loosen up and focus on your meditation practice. The more pressure you put on yourself, the more difficult it will be to break free from your physical body. Relax to become light. You will be able to transcend into a higher realm of awareness once you have become light enough. Thus, the key to successful meditation is to relax and let go.

You Are Safe

One thing you should be aware of is that meditation is a risk-free activity. Unfortunately, some individuals believe that meditation may put you in danger. You're okay as long as you don't meditate while driving, crossing the street, or in comparable situations. In reality, meditators and gurus have reported that you will be promptly returned to your physical body if you are put in danger while you are meditating. So, while you meditate, you should not be concerned about your safety as it will only split your efforts and focus. Instead, devote all of your attention to your meditation practice.

It is best to only teach you the most necessary instructions when meditating, as having too much knowledge might cause your mind to wander even more. It is now time for you to discover and experience what meditation genuinely entails. Do not be disheartened if you don't observe any changes, even in your state of mind. You will improve as long as you practice regularly. Let us now proceed to the meditation itself.

Meditation Practice for Beginners

It is an excellent idea to learn about meditation with the breath, or simply breathing meditation, for your first meditation. This is the most fundamental meditation practice in the world. Do not, however, underestimate the effectiveness of this meditation. Many spiritual teachers, including the great Buddha, practiced this meditation for a long time. It is also not unusual for seasoned monks to practice this meditation for years. The simplicity of this meditation is its strength. The procedure is as follows:

Take a contemplative stance. Simply unwind and don't think about anything. Now concentrate on your breathing. Gently inhale and exhale. In... Out... Do you comprehend how delicate life is? This in-and-out breathing rhythm absolutely cannot be disrupted, or else there will be a danger or death. Consider the beauty of your breath. Take a deep breath in and a deep breath out. Take a look at the gift of life. Concentrate solely on your breathing at this point. Concentrate solely on your breathing, and don't think about anything else. Let go and relax. Make a connection with your breath.

This meditation method can be practiced for as long as you like. If you're just getting started, you might only want to do it for a few minutes. However, it is worth noting that many skilled meditators use this for an extended amount of time, even hours. For the time being, simply do whatever seems right to you. It's not a good idea to hasten your spiritual development. Just remember to constantly give it your all and be devoted to it. It should also be noted that this simple meditation energizes and strengthens all of your chakras. Regular practice of this meditation will enable you to achieve a state of consciousness that you have never previously experienced. You will be in a serene and harmonious state by the end of this meditation.

Common Errors

Let us now discuss the most prevalent faults or errors in meditation. It is good to be aware of these hazards to avoid them. However, it should be highlighted that many of these errors are difficult to avoid, so do not be disappointed if you find yourself doing them after having been warned. Simply do your best and keep practicing.

Thinking

You should recognize that meditation is more about doing than thinking. It is not about thinking about the current moment but being in it. When you meditate, don't think about anything; simply be.

Another typical blunder is to ask yourself, "Am I doing it right?" while meditating. If you consider this, you are going about it incorrectly. This type of inquiry should be asked after the meditation rather than during the meditation itself. When you meditate, you should not split yourself in any manner.

Incorrect Focus

It's true that when you meditate, you usually have to concentrate on something. Unfortunately, some meditators find themselves focused on focusing rather than the purpose of an object in meditation. Okay, this may be a little complex, but you must comprehend this lesson.

When you meditate, don't tell yourself that you need to concentrate on this or that. Instead, you must do it. Concentrating requires action, not just a directive. There is a distinction between genuinely concentrating on your breathing and telling yourself that you should focus on your breathing. You should take some time to think about this and ensure that you fully comprehend it.

Scratching

When you meditate, you may notice that a section of your body becomes itchy. Of course, the instinct is to scratch it. The difficulty is that the mind's attention will be drawn back to the physical body. If you keep doing this, you will never be able to enter a trance or a deeper state of awareness.

So, what are your options? You'll simply have to ignore it. Although it is natural to experience itching when meditating, you should not allow it to upset or distract you. This may be tough to accomplish at first, but you have to fight it and become used to it. You will no longer be disturbed by this irritating sensation after enough practice. You won't even consider it. Remember to simply ignore it. The more you think about it, the more it will distract you. Once again, consistent practice is essential.

Inadequate Practice

Learning to meditate is similar to picking up a new skill. It also takes practice, much like mastering a new skill. Do not expect to do well if you only practice once a week. If you are serious about spiritual growth, you should make it a point to meditate at least once a day. If you're just getting started, you may perform as little as five or ten minutes of meditation every day. However, as you develop and become more accustomed to it, you will need to practice more. Continuous practice is essential. It is recommended that you establish a meditation schedule and stick to it. In this manner, you can ensure that you set aside time for meditation. It is difficult to achieve an elevated level of spiritual growth without consistent practice.

Falling Asleep

This is a typical blunder made by newcomers. The good news is that it is preventable. There are a few things you should keep in mind. If falling asleep is a problem for you, you should avoid meditating in a lying-down position, as this is the posture that will most probably cause you to fall asleep. You may also consider meditating somewhere other than your bed. The bed signals to the mind that it is time to relax or sleep. As a result, meditating on your bed may indicate to your brain that it is time to sleep rather than meditate. Again, the sitting position is the optimum posture. Second, do not meditate if you are fatigued. Falling asleep is simpler when you are exhausted. Third, do not meditate before going to bed. Many novices who meditate before going to bed fall asleep entirely. This is because you would be exhausted and tired by this point. Instead, you can meditate first thing in the morning.

Of course, if you don't have trouble falling asleep while meditating, you can skip these precautions. In that case, you are free to meditate at any time of day or night. What matters most is that you figure out what works best for you.

However, don't be too hard on yourself. If you fall asleep despite taking the precautions mentioned above, it is most likely because you needed the rest, so try again some other time.

Having Expectations

When you meditate, you must focus your full attention on your meditation target. This also implies that you must let go of any expectations. Expecting anything to happen, whether this or that, will simply split your energies. Expectations will also prevent you from giving your full attention. Instead of setting expectations, simply relax and continue with your meditation practice.

Being Too Critical of Yourself

You should not be too hard on yourself. Even if you believe you cannot meditate effectively, be kind to yourself. Being irritated will only undermine your efforts. Instead of being harsh on yourself, try to relax and think about the situation thoughtfully and kindly. Find out what mistakes you've been making and make the necessary changes to remedy them. When you are cheerful or full of positive energy, you will be able to meditate more efficiently. Instead of putting pressure on yourself, which isn't even helpful for you, channel that energy towards focusing harder on your practice and giving it your all. Keep in mind that even if you give it your all, you should not expect to be enlightened or activate your Kundalini straight away. This requires a significant amount of practice, time, and effort. Instead, acknowledge that you are on the correct road and are well to mastery.

Otherworldly Bypassing

Otherworldly bypassing is the phase at which we employ otherworldliness to detour us from feeling we will need to return to. This makes our training less practical and eases down our otherworldly development. However, it might feel amazing for the time being.

How may we forestall bypassing?

Be sure that you are centered and focused on your body as you practice. In case you're having a lot of an 'up and out' of body understanding, you may not be anchored enough and are uncomfortable detouring an area, companion to your sensations, and enable your training to encompass them, not get away from them.

Different Approaches

You might inevitably compare the time you spend meditating to the time you spend driving, cleaning dishes, planting, or even working. You may realize that you are spending a lot of time meditating, even if you only planned to do so for one hour. Don't feel like you have to shorten the amount of time you spend meditating; instead, set aside at least one hour every day to meditate without interruptions. You can set an alarm to let you know when your specified time is almost up. After some time, the appropriate practice expands in phases like a dream experience. You need enough time to let go of your thoughts and delve into the essence of who you are, forgetting the world's chaos. Alternatively, you could move at every 15-minute increment of your meditation, which might provide extra motivation to keep going.

Failure to Start

Meditation works better when you do it. The best practice is the one you follow. We may have the best intentions for making time for training, but how often do we find a viable pace? There's a technique for 'getting in the vessel,' which will make you feel so good that you'll want to keep going. Declare to yourself that you will only sit for two minutes and then find a feasible speed; minutes will feel better regardless of whether you achieve a feasible speed. When you speak your plans out loud, your sensory system will feel the effects, and you'll need to do it. Reflection is usually more relaxing and peaceful than sleep. Use this trick to stay connected to your daily training.

Gimmicky Versions

There exist several innovative, minor deviations from traditional meditation. The approach can be negatively affected if there are many of them. I'm not claiming that only old ideas are viable. It is, however, a part of what I'm saying. Experts who lack comprehensive otherworldly training believe that reinventing the wheel is superior to anything else create many innovative yet gimmicky frameworks. Remember that traditional schools of activity have a substantial number, if not a significant amount, of experience promoting reflection and observing understudies improv via instruction. Even though two hundred years of modern science has a lot to offer, considerable progress is an ancient passion. Gimmicky versions of meditation can attract our attention and help us focus on the significance of brain preparation, but as a real professional, be careful in practicing these deviations from ancient research.

Being a Teacher

Some people are sensitive to this one. Imagine you're a teacher. We benefit from exceptional trainers in areas where we need to exceed expectations. The same can be said for otherworldliness. A meditation teacher can help you smooth out any rough spots in your practice, making it more spectacular and powerful while also assisting you in avoiding simple blunders. After some time, as you and your training evolve, a skilled instructor may help alter the training to best suit your current stage of growth, much to how a good golf trainer employs different tactics at various stages of a player's development. Regardless, don't allow con artists to keep you from seeking a qualified and reputable master. Keep a lookout for those dressed as such who are more interested in benefits for themselves. It can make an enormous impact on your growth and awakening.

Day vs. Night

It is acceptable to stop and reflect during the day. It may be beneficial to meditate early morning and late at night. There's a reason so many priests get up in the middle of the night to practice. It's serene, nothing is going on, and there's nothing much to do. You can meditate for an extended period without being interrupted.

Similarly, contemplating at 3 a.m. has a different mood than working on anything during the day. You'll notice how your body absorbs the vibrancy and motion of your surroundings. Early morning and late-night meditations encourage more significant internal and external movement than daytime thinking. The dead of night is also an exceptionally enchanting time to practice.

Using Too Many Props

A few items can assist specialists in focusing. However, be wary of relying too heavily on them. The goal of introspection is to become at ease with oneself, to be content with one's own inner experience of life. Thus, it may be useful to sit and confront yourself in the same way you came into this world: with nothing. A plethora of items may detract from your core nature experience. Some people, for example, have a cushion, beads, sacred water, a raised place, a flame, another person, and so on. The problem is practicing can become difficult unless they have those items. Two or three props to help you stay awake or focused may be part of your training but consider minimizing them if they aren't necessary. Try thinking without any distractions, music, or anything else.

Relying on Guided Meditations

Guided meditation might help some people connect with their internal selves and access the peaceful place inside of them. However, you may not want to rely on them every time you practice. Meditation helps you connect with yourself. It might become a brace when we rely too heavily on someone else to guide us through an event. There's nothing wrong with having an experienced co-pilot fly the plane with you, but it's better to try out the controls and learn how to fly it yourself. A combination of self and guided meditation can provide the best of both worlds.

Not Expanding Your Practice

Regarding the significance of full-length formal preparation, accepting that this is business as usual necessitates broadening your meditation to include various aspects of the day. Meditation is an all-weather task that can be completed whenever and wherever you want. The long-term goal is to live in meditation to bridge the gap between training and non-practice. Try keeping your eyes open during a conversation or while working on occasion. It's a mistake to limit your unearthly relationship to the events you mark on your calendar.

CHAPTER 6: KUNDALINI EXERCISES

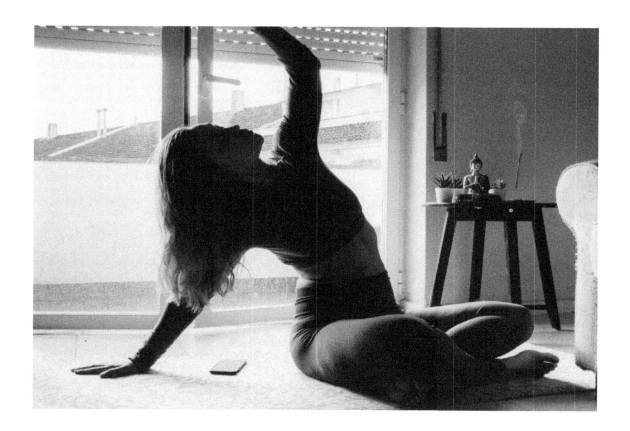

Kundalini and Chi's Connection

Prana is also known as chi. Many words are used to describe Prana, depending on the culture or area. Prana is chi in China, pneuma in Greece, and mana in ancient Polynesia. In India, Prana is a word that is commonly used. Nonetheless, all of these words relate to the same energy. As previously said, chi is different from Kundalini for the reasons previously indicated.

Kundalini Yoga's Health Advantages

The Kundalini Awakening has been linked to a variety of health advantages. It supports good health in several ways: It controls and corrects blood pressure, is an excellent stress reliever, and can fight and even cure diabetes and other disorders. It also has many other health advantages, including relief from stomach and liver disorders, kidney stones, and gallstones difficulties. Some even say that waking the Kundalini may treat significant ailments such as cancer. Indeed, as you feel the power that pours through your body when your Kundalini awakens, you realize that everything is possible. Clear thinking is a frequent effect of Kundalini's awakening, as is greater concentration, attentiveness, and mental power.

It is also worth mentioning that many of these advantages may be obtained even if your Kundalini is not fully awakened. As you will see from this book, the various practices can provide many health advantages. Of course, if you want to reap all of the benefits, you must first activate your Kundalini.

Various Kundalini Meditations and Exercises

It should be highlighted that no one workout or meditation practice would ensure Kundalini activation. For this to happen, accumulative spiritual practices and spiritual development are required. All of the exercises in this book will assist you in awakening your Kundalini. However, keep in mind that learning isn't enough. You must also put that information into a practical and ongoing practice.

You may be wondering why this book is so dense with mental and meditation practices. This is because waking the Kundalini requires greater mental effort and practice. You should anticipate spending a lot of time meditating. There are, however, physical activities that might help you activate the Kundalini. Any type of physical activity is a natural means of purifying the body of bad energy. You may engage in physical activity or exercise depending on your fitness level. To begin, you might wish to do some walking exercises. You can go for a jog or a decent run if you feel fit and healthy. Exercising is, of course, beneficial to the physical body.

Meditation is the most effective approach to activate the Kundalini. You will discover several meditation techniques as you read this book. Some of these meditation practices will directly boost and activate your Kundalini, while others may do so indirectly. However, it is worth mentioning that all meditation activities aid in the rising of the Kundalini. As a result, you may be assured that no effort will ever be in vain.

Kundalini Activation's Impact on the Body, Emotions, and Psyche

As previously stated, awakening the Kundalini provides several advantages to the physical body. It will help you feel more centered and peaceful in terms of emotions. Even before you reach the point of waking, you will benefit from its favorable emotional impacts. You'll feel less anxious and more in command of yourself and your emotions.

In terms of thinking, you will have greater mental clarity. You will be able to think and evaluate things more clearly. It will provide you with clarity that you have never had before. Having such mental clarity is equivalent to having full peace of mind.

How Kundalini Feels

You might not feel anything if your Kundalini is still latent. Moreover, the more you practice on your Kundalini, the more you will be able to feel it, mainly when you undertake meditation techniques that directly activate the Kundalini. You may expect a huge energy flow through your body when Kundalini awakens.

The sensation is frequently described as warm, as energy is typically warm. It's also a wonderful way to unwind. It is even said to be more enjoyable than having an orgasm. It's a spiritual ecstasy, you could say.

How to Remove the Impediments that Impede Kundalini from Ascending Smoothly

Blockages can inhibit the Kundalini from waking and ascending. To prevent this, you must ensure that energy flows freely via the energy pathways' meridians. You should also keep your chakras cleaned and aligned. Don't worry; you'll find out how to accomplish it later in the book.

What, though, is the source of these snarls? A variety of factors can cause blocked drains. Excessive stress is a typical cause of this. Being stressed has become increasingly prevalent in today's society, which is a shame since it implies that many individuals do not have a free energy flow. If you wish to awaken your Kundalini, you must ensure that your stress levels are managed. It should be remembered that stress is not inherently harmful; when you fail to manage it appropriately, it becomes harmful. Several more factors might obstruct the free flow of energy, such as negative experiences, emotional breakdowns, psychic attacks, etc. When addressing blockages, it is critical to identify the root source of the problem. A typical error is to treat a blockage without addressing the underlying reason. As a result, if a blockage is caused by work-related stress, you must make some changes at work. You can't merely treat the consequence or the result without addressing the cause.

As a result, any obstructions or healing should be performed on two levels: physical and spiritual. You may need to make some lifestyle modifications on a physical level. You must practice the meditations explained in depth later in the book on a spiritual level.

How to Awaken a Dormant Kundalini

As previously said, there is no single guideline or practice that may ensure Kundalini's awakening. This will have to be determined by your general spiritual growth and practices. However, there are two methods to awaken a dormant Kundalini: on your own or with the assistance of a spiritual teacher.

This book is all about being able to accomplish it on your own. If you want to achieve it with the guidance of a spiritual master or guru, you must be completely dedicated and submit to your master. Your teacher may also ask you to engage in particular meditation techniques; nevertheless, some individuals claim to be able to awaken one's Kundalini as long as the student surrenders all and submits to their master. The issue here is that finding a true master is difficult. Unfortunately, many people profess to be masters but are shams and hackers. Another issue with this technique is that while a master may be able to activate your Kundalini, your soul may not be prepared. This is about your spiritual growth. As a result, when it comes to the Kundalini Awakening, it is highly encouraged that you perform the work yourself so that your soul can grow and prepare you for it. Of course, you are allowed to seek assistance from a master but do not disregard your spiritual development.

It's reasonable to presume your Kundalini is dormant right now, which explains why you're reading this book. Do not be concerned; this book will guide you and teach you the procedures necessary to awaken the twisting force. Simply remain with me so you may learn as you accompany me on this road of authentic Kundalini Awakening.

Spine Flexibility Maintenance

To introduce someone to Kundalini Yoga (KY), it is vital to preserve the spine and ensure a healthy body in compliance. According to yogis, an individual's spine flexibility defines their youth.

The most prevalent complaint among individuals as they age is discomfort in their lower backs and upper backs, between their shoulders. As a result, it makes sense that regularly taking care of your spine will be critical in avoiding much of your back discomfort. Unfortunately, there is no quick remedy for back pain, but this series of exercises will be an excellent maintenance program for your spine and, thus, your back.

Beginning

Sit quietly in a low-key setting. Concentrate on just being present with your breath. Slow down your breathing and take deep breaths from your abdomen. Concentrate and become one with your body's sensations. Feel for and tune in to your beat.

Allowing yourself a few minutes to simply "be" will enable you to settle down, become grounded, and create your own space.

Getting Tuned In

Chanting the "ADI MANTRA" might help you get tuned in and concentrated from the start when practicing Kundalini Yoga.

Exercises

Rotations of the Pelvis

- Simple pose
- Place hands on your knees
- Roll the pelvis around deeply with a grinding action
- Relax and be in the moment
- To create a movement meditation, perform this exercise for 1-2 minutes, or approximately 26 rotations in each direction

Spinal Flexion (Spinal Flex)

- Simple posture
- Grasp ankles
- Inhale deeply as you flex your spine forward
- Keep your shoulders relaxed and your head straight (no up and down head movements)

- Exhale. Relax your spine
- Continue rhythmically, taking deep breaths
- Feel the energy flowing down your spine as you inhale
- Notice your exhales returning to your Third Eye
- On the inhale, mentally vibrate Sat, and on the exhale, mentally vibrate Nam.
- Repeat this exercise 100 times or for 1-3 minutes

Neck Rolls

- Sit with your back straight, yet relaxed
- Move the head back slightly to place it directly on the spine
- Slightly lower the chin
- Roll the neck slowly in one direction
- Roll the neck in the other direction
- Use the head's weight to move it around
- During these neck rolls, be exceedingly meticulous to gradually work out the tight regions and areas with higher tension
- Do this for at least one minute in each direction
- After that, sit quietly and become one with your body and spine feelings
- Advantages: Reduces neck strain and stimulates the thyroid

Shoulder Shrugs

- Relaxed position or sitting on heels
- Shrug both shoulders up on the inhale
- Exhale by lowering your shoulders
- Continue doing this exercise for 1-2 minutes
- Advantages: Reduces shoulder strain and soothes the upper back

Side Twists

- Sit on heels
- Place your hands on your shoulders, fingers in front, and thumb in back
- Exhale, then twist left
- Exhale and then twist right
- Twist the head to each side, as well
- With each twist, you should notice a progressive increase in rotation in your spine
- Keep your elbows parallel to the ground

- Allow the arms to swing freely along with the body
- It can also be done while standing
- Repeat 26 times or for 1 to 2 minutes
- Following that, inhale center, hold your breath, the root lock, exhale, and feel the energy circulate, calming you
- Advantages: opens the heart and promotes the upper spine

Bends on the Side

- Simple posture
- Venus lock fingers (clasp hands behind the neck with interlaced fingers)
- Bend sideways, keeping your back straight
- Point the elbow toward the floor, keeping it beside the hip
- Inhale, then bend left
- Exhale and bend right
- Sit back and unwind (not an arched but a controlled spine)
- Only sway sideways
- It is possible to perform this exercise while standing
- Repeat up to 26 times or for 1 to 2 minutes
- Advantages: Stimulates the liver and intestines while increasing spine flexibility

Cobra

- Lie down on the floor
- Place your palms on the floor beneath your shoulders
- As you inhale, slowly arch your back upwards
- Begin with the nose, then the chin
- Push off with your hands, vertebrae by vertebrae, until you are as arched as possible while avoiding lower back tension
- Emphasize proper stretching
- Extend from the heart center upwards
- Fire Breath — take long, deep breaths
- Continue for another 2 to 3 minutes
- Following that, inhale, hold, bring the energy up the spine, and root lock
- Exhale one vertebra at a time as you come down
- Take a moment to unwind for 1 to 3 minutes

- Advantages: Strengthens the lower back, relieves back strain, and regulates the flow of sexual and naval energy

Leg Stretch (Alternating)

- Legs spread wide apart
- While keeping your knees straight, grip your toes (or anyplace comfortable or possible to grasp without bending knees)
- Inhale center
- Exhale downward toward your left leg
- Inhale center
- Exhale downward toward your right leg
- To expand the pelvis, move from the hips rather than the waist
- Maintain a straight spine (comfortably) while stretching your back
- Stretch muscles without straining
- Breathe deeply for 1 to 2 minutes more
- Then, inhale center, hold breath, apply root lock, and relax. Bring your legs back together, bouncing up and down a few times to relax your muscles, and massage your muscles if necessary
- Advantages: opens up the pelvis and expands the leg muscles

CHAPTER 7: YOGA POSES OF KUNDALINI

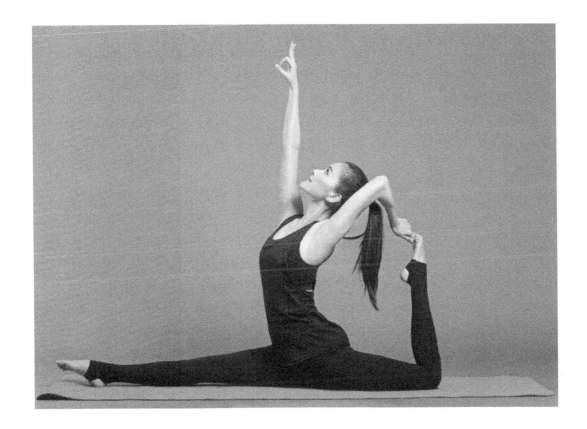

Each Kundalini yoga practice (asana) is performed in tandem with a specific inhaling and exhaling method that amplifies the benefits of the postures while harnessing liberating energy in the lower system and enabling it to ascend. Kundalini sequences may comprise quick, repeated motions performed in tandem with the defined breathing methods or holding a stance while inhaling precisely. When you deeply inhale and exhale, you will notice that a breath comes in and goes out simultaneously. When you become aware of your intake and exhale, you realize that you are distinct from your physical body, but so is your breath. Then you know you're only a spectator, detached from both the physical body and the breathing process. Inhaling and exhaling might help you identify your dissociation from your body.

Meditation is similar to opening the entryway of your dark house to let the sun in. Even when the sun rises in the east, you will be in the dark if you keep your doors closed.

The simplest way to begin meditation is to engage the transition during a time of extremes. Every change occurs when extremes are reached. The shift occurs when your sensations reach extremes.

Millions of stressors are held in your body that you are unaware of, even if they may result from your actions. Society has produced an uncomfortable way of life in which we are expected to smile even when we are upset. Because of these societal constraints, your body has become a storage facility for tensions; thousands of tensions have gathered within your body. These types of conflicts need to be aired and resolved. However, it is seldom permitted to vent these repressed frustrations physically. However, your body may become as delicate as flowery with the release of tensions, knots, and complexes.

Yoga and meditation practices can have a variety of physical effects. Several physical ailments may disappear, vitality may rise, and numerous material changes occur within our bodies. Several non-active glands throughout the body can become active. The whole chemistry of the human body can undergo a sea of alterations. Our bodies begin to interpret, believe, and realize the current circumstance as entirely new. All of the body's electric circuits start to alter and change. The body has a certain amount of carbon dioxide and oxygen; contemplative breathing alters this ratio. As soon as this ratio shifts, changes in the body, mind, blood, and central nervous system will follow.

When we plant a seedling, it takes time to develop into a sprout. Similarly, as a seed, you will take time to crumble and dissolve, while sprouting occurs instantly.

Accept everything that happens to you and let go of yourself completely, accepting that everything happens independently. Meditation is a technique for restoring one's normalcy and healing dynamics. This existence energy descends when you enter the body and ascends when you enter meditation. During meditation, deep and fast breathing hammers and relocates its placement in the center. If your mind is overwhelmed with any lusty urge related to wrath or desire, slow down your inhalation, unwind, and it will leave you. This energy cannot operate until it is activated merely by breathing. Nobody can be upset if they continue to inhale slowly, regularly, and relaxedly. Deep breathing reaches the base center (near Kundalini), and as the experience progresses, you will comprehend the exact speed necessary merely by inhaling.

Deep Breathing —- 30 Minutes in the Morning

Stage 1 (10 Minutes)

Sit down and retain your distance from others so that folks who want to lie down can do so freely. There should be silence, and no one should talk. Close your eyes and start inhaling deeply. Inhale as much as you can and expel as much as you can. Inhale and exhale with all of your force; breathe and exhale deeply.

Apply yourself thoroughly, and within the first 10 minutes, focus ceaselessly while deep breathing.

Allow each fiber of the body to vibrate in unison while breathing and exhaling. Also, make sure you're breathing thoroughly. Continue to observe the air moving out and coming in regularly. From inside, notice how your breathing is coming in and going out at a constant and rapid speed. The deep inhalation will start to awaken energy inside you. A sleeping light within you will begin to shine due to your strong inhaling and exhaling.

Stage 2 (10 Minutes)

Entirely disregard your body and relax. Deeply inhale and exhale, then release your body. Continue breathing for 10 minutes. Allow the body to assume certain postures and gestures if they occur. Breathing should not be slowed. Allow whatever happens in your body to happen; don't get in the way of it.

As the energy level rises, inhale and exhale deeply. Then, let the body be free and unfettered. Allow yourself to let go of your body, and don't be afraid to feel your emotions; allow them to come and wash away.

Stage 3 (10 Minutes)

Continue breathing deeply. Add the mental projection for the recommendation to enter meditation. "I want to enter meditation," you say to yourself. Allow this desire to pervade every breath you take: "I wish to enter into meditation." The more you exert yourself, the more rest you will have. The worse the storm, the deeper the meditation will sink into you. "I wish to enter into meditation." Let every beat of your heart desire. Allow whatever occurs to the body to happen as it will. After that, abandon all attempts at breathing exercises and reach the last stage of relaxation. Give up everything and lie in wait for a sight of an entry into meditation for 10 minutes. Now, softly open your eyes and breathe deeply but slowly; gradually rise.

It is pleasant to be able to be anything you choose just by letting your attention and latent energies of the body amass and work with you. There is undoubtedly endless energy (Kundalini) hidden inside all humans, but we have never utilized this energy in a meaningful way. We have not activated all of the roots inside our existence, so we encounter obstacles.

Daily meditation will eventually allow Kundalini to connect the students with the divine power, and that connection will develop deeper and more joyful as the disciples practice deep breathing.

Process of the Mind

The brain is undoubtedly always looking and constantly desiring something. The true object lies in the future; it has nothing to do with the present. The actual mind requires the potential to shift or move in the past or future. It would not occupy the present; there is no room for it. All meditation/yoga approaches change the mind's focus from the past or future to the present now. It is no longer there once ideas arrive at the present instant. Ideas and thoughts come to a halt and are unable to progress.

Meditation tends to blur the lines between what is good and evil. According to meditation, dividing is impure, while not dividing is pure. To a youngster, the division has no significance. The small youngster is not aware of any distinction between good and evil. That unawareness is innocence. The more the child's thinking grows, the more unclean they will become. Because the mind is constantly evolving, everything will eventually become impure. Meditation/yoga guarantees that when a person reverts to the state of a kid, that person will become pure. Finally, innocence is reclaimed. However, you now comprehend the full body as well as the consciousness.

Meditation allows you to think with your good inner nature, thinking that many individuals are born great, and that goodness is their character.

Natural growth is required; an individual does not require every imposition. This is the leading cause; therefore, why is nothing considered flawed?

"You cannot enter my Kingdom of God until you become like children," Jesus declared. Jesus has enjoyed both darkness and light, but now he has transcended both. Life and death, love and hatred, and good and evil are all aspects of one unified and tangible event. Jesus believed in the inherent goodness of every person.

Every one of the energies within you has been certified by meditation science. The objective is to bring about a transformation, not to erase anything. The first stage is to acquire an accepting attitude. Whatever activities you take, they are only on the outskirts of your existence; at heart, everyone remains good. Man has a center, yet he typically lives apart from it. Throughout, this develops latent enmity and continual suffering. Being out of balance may lead to many mental worries and unhealthy sexual life.

Anger might feel like insanity at times, but it is not permanent. You may be able to recover from this event. When you are peaceful, you may be able to touch the core, resulting in a joyful but fleeting experience. The delightful moment you are experiencing has truly migrated to the basic center. We'll keep moving between these two, but it'll be perilous this time since you'll see a moving picture of yourself.

Desire typically grows, and everything you acquire becomes useless; it is useless the instant you obtain it. This is wanted, and there is no resolution.

When someone takes all, you are in its entirety, coming to a halt. There is no concern because stress cannot exist at such a time.

This non-desiring mind has been the brain focused inside the self. Buddha lives in the present moment, whereas the maniac is the polar opposite. We reside somewhere between these two extremes of existence. It might happen when thoughts halt or when there is a brief period of no desire. Love is desireless; you might want love, but true love is always desireless. When love occurs, there is no wish; the mind is peaceful, serene, and comfortable. However, these types of occurrences are rare.

You may be at peace with yourself, and this special pleasure fills you like an encompassing aroma. That is the primary cause, but why does love drastically alter someone? For a few seconds, you are exactly like Buddha when you are in a state of love. The experience will not last long since your mind will interfere with the mechanism. You don't learn how to exist if you don't have a desire. These experiences are unique to each individual and cannot be replicated.

Indications when the Kundalini Yoga Suits You

Every person uniquely experiences the world; thus, you are unquestionably unique. The real feeling would be the same, but the observer behind all of these would be different. Everything that causes tensions and disputes starts to fade. You feel that a new life is coming to you; you are getting unburdened. You have the impression that you have grown to be weightless. Everything you do today will be different. This type of distinction may be seen everywhere. Soon, a new source of energy (Kundalini) becomes available, which is significantly greater than our fundamental life energy.

The cosmos is the crystallization of energy, and life is the extension of that energy. The change of energy is the sensation of awareness. The entire cosmos is a manifestation of the same energy in infinite forms. Our existence would be meaningless if we did not pose such fundamental issues. Our inner vision is not as huge as a mountain; it is merely a thin layer of dirt that blocks and conceals all of life's genuine facts. We all long to get in touch with this realm of wonder and pleasure, yet it looks like nothing more than hollow rhetoric.

There is a core within us, but it remains inert and inactive if the life force does not reach there. Kundalini yoga involves always obtaining life force from the center so that the bloom may quickly bud, and the light can easily begin to burn.

Every seed has the right to grow into a tree, but they do not always do so. The seed can grow into a tree, but it must be planted and dissolved into the soil before growing into a tree. That seed only grows into a tree when it is ready to be buried.

Each child has an unlimited number of opportunities, but no one can readily explain or verify the existence of these options. A river cannot become an ocean, yet it admires the ocean. There is only one way to take a leap of faith without knowing the consequences; the leap must be daring.

The sixth sense, or Third Eye, is located in the mind. This center is locked and inert, but once activated, we should be able to see life in several dimensions. The life force resides within us, yet it cannot manifest until it reaches that core, allowing the manifestation to occur. The location where life energy is stored is similar to a pool at the navel (Kundalini). Life extends in all directions from here.

If you are ready for the new, you must muster the guts to be a part of the old. New centers will awaken, a new personality will form, and new experiences may occur; everything will be unique.

In meditation, completely release yourself, as if you were a guy letting go at the river's mercy and then floating with its stream. Higher powers have seized control. We no longer need to be concerned; all we need to do is go.

The small energy that we all store throughout a night's sleep depletes as soon as we get out of bed each day. We have no notion how to conserve a significant amount of energy daily. Meditation requires a lot of energy, and if you don't preserve it, you'll grow tired. A small amount of energy is saved at night, so you feel refreshed. If you accept everything and enjoy it, you will eliminate the need for any form of complaint throughout your life. You will then realize how serene and joyful life can be when you are not grudging. All of the yogic postures were discovered at various levels of meditation. In the state of meditation, our bodies assumed numerous positions, which were known as yogic postures. There is a connection between the body and the mind. When the body is in a given posture, the reason will follow suit by entering a similar state. Our bodies have their methods of expressing themselves in various levels of meditation.

If, during meditation, your body begins to bend and twist in a certain way, and you try to stop it, you may disrupt its specific inner state and advancement. If you have suppressed tears, they will come to the surface during meditation. If you have been hiding your laughter, it will come out. Allow things to happen, and then allow them to be washed away.

Matter and mind are not two distinct problems. What we call matter is consciousness asleep, and what we call awareness is consciousness awakened. Matter and mind are two separate aspects of the same entity. Science discovered that the only thing that exists is energy after extensive research. When spirituality dug deep, it found that only the soul exists and that the soul is energy. Consciousness is matters while it is asleep, and consciousness is when it is woken.

Meditation is a way of entering this eternal moment. When time runs out, one is admitted to meditation. It occurs between two points: when one instant has passed, and the next moment has yet to arrive. It takes place between two points in time.

Your sorrow is measured by the passage of time. The more dissatisfied you are, the longer time will pass. Misery is similar to a character in that it looks eternal; it appears as though it will never cease. Anguish lengthens time, while joy shortens it. In meditation, time ceases to exist.

The specific waves of ideas prevent the mind from reflecting. Knowledge is attained in a state of consciousness in which everything is silent and motionless, and just the knowledge remains. The stillness of mind is required to realize knowledge, but nothing more is required once learned.

False impressions are no longer possible if a glimpse of truth is available. While the possibility of a mistaken impression remains, everything inside of us remains steady and tranquil.

Before beginning meditation, all thoughts, feelings, and desires must come to a halt. The thirst and longing for the Supreme have been with all humans. The vast majority of individuals we live with are utterly bereft of this drive. A desire for money or fame drives the majority of those around you. Our society's focus is to want money or fame, so the genuine desire for the Supreme is suppressed. When heavenly hunger appears, all aspirations for money and glory go.

It is a delusion that humans are "doers," and this idea causes individuals to be dissatisfied and wretched. It is only a fantasy that man is a doer; if this desire fades, you will be able to enter meditation and awaken Kundalini. The funniest aspect of dreaming is that it is entirely true. Illusions are generated in this manner, but they will not progress to the path of Meditation.

Initial Benefits of Kundalini Yoga

Many physical and natural disorders impede and complicate our everyday lives. However, by practicing Kundalini Yoga, we can begin to see these ailments go away and our longevity grow. An unhealthy sexual life and anxiety are caused by past societal teachings and large energy knots. These knots will be freed up for the calming procedure.

Your face will regain a huge and astonishing radiance, and your facial expression will become gorgeous. It will emerge from refining the many auras contained inside the seven bodies.

New sensory organs will be awakened inside you, and certain previously dormant glands within your system may be reactivated. You will be able to cleanse the physical body, which will improve the DNA activation process. At the time of DNA make-up activations, impulsive healings can occur. These are usually associated with severe physical and mental problems.

Following your actions, a cleansing technique begins to purify your physical, emotional, and mental bodies. You might be able to enter the etheric body, which is the emotional body and the first step toward achievement in the science of meditation. As a result, you may have many subtle experiences and will begin to sense the usable (etheric) world of Devas (positive energies) as well as Pretas (negative energies).

Kundalini Awakening is exceedingly harmful if the followers have not acquired the purity of body, mind, and emotions. It may cause high fever and spinal discomfort. To begin Kundalini yoga, you must follow the correct recommendations for a yoga professional.

Many followers have had encounters with folks who have experimented with an unaware or unapproved technique. In such cases, the first chakra (Muladhar), which preserves Kundalini's purity, the base chakra, responds to the breach by creating a wave of heat. The student may lose control of their body and thoughts in this circumstance. During the Kundalini energy awakening, the disciple's face becomes luminous. The disciple seems much younger, and their physique becomes more dynamic and well-proportioned. The disciple's entire demeanor transforms into something beautiful and captivating, and they can progress further.

Kundalini Yoga vs. Other Types of Yoga

Several yoga practices have various names, offering the mind, body, and spirit advantages. To help you understand how Kundalini differs from other popular yoga practices, below is a broad review of some of the yoga types being performed.

- Hatha Yoga – In general, Hatha is a broad word that refers to various positions often utilized in different yoga practices. It is a blend of breathing and strength-building exercise that promotes physical vitality.
- Ashtanga Yoga – Ashtanga is a Sanskrit word that means "eight-limb way." It is a physically challenging sequence of poses designed for the more experienced yoga practitioner.
- Vinyasa Yoga – Vinyasa is a Sanskrit term that means "to put in a specific way." It is a more athletic, faster-paced variation of Ashtanga yoga that uses breath and movement to connect mind and body while developing flexibility.
- Iyengar Yoga – This yoga focuses on alignment via slow, precise movement and breath control. It makes minimal modifications and uses a variety of props to improve posture and form — deeper and more unwinding.
- Bikram Yoga – Bikram, sometimes known as "hot yoga," has become a craze. It is a series of yoga positions performed twice in a hot, sauna-like chamber with 105 percent and 40 percent humidity levels.

- Yin Yoga – The term Yin relates to the heavenly feminine notion. This yoga is slow and sitting for most of the practice, with postures or stretches sustained for extended periods, up to 2-4 minutes. This yoga technique encourages mental relaxation and inner serenity.
- Jivamukti Yoga – It is based on a Vinyasa style flow and combines chanting and deeper Hindu spiritual instruction. It encourages a connection to Mother Earth and being a living person on her.

There are many more yoga styles and practices to explore, but this is an excellent introduction to some of the most frequent and popular varieties practiced in the West. Many of them are directly taken from Eastern yoga philosophy. In contrast, various gurus and yogis have changed others to foster new ways of learning and connection to mind, body, and spirit.

So, what distinguishes Kundalini Yoga from the other yoga practices? Like Hatha and certain different yoga types, Kundalini yoga focuses on asanas (postures) and Pranayama (breath). Because Kundalini aims to awaken the latent, pure awareness energy, there is an added emphasis on what is known as the "subtle body." The term "subtle body" refers to the light inside or the electromagnetic field within and around us. This emphasis is not only on the physical self, but it also claims that by awakening the subtle body and cleansing it through awakening, you can heal both the physical and spiritual selves.

The following methods would be included in a regular Kundalini yoga practice:

- Meditation – Mental focus to alleviate stress and anxiety or boost energy and open chakras
- Pranayama – Meditation and energy movement through breath control or breath extensions
- Asanas – A body posture or pose used for exercise and meditation, including reclining, standing, inverted, twisting, balancing, and seated stances
- Bandha – A muscle group, locking to boost pranic energy to remove poisons or impurities in the body
- Mantra – Sanskrit words or phrases thought to have a mental and spiritual impact when uttered or chanted following the breath and/or posture.
- Mudra – A symbolic hand positioning with a spiritual meaning that elicits energy control and redistribution throughout the being.
- Kriya – A physical manifestation of activated Kundalini intended to produce a specific outcome (Ex: spontaneous body movement; trance-like states of consciousness; involuntary tremors, shaking, or tingling all over the body; change in body odor); It can also refer to the effort expended in conducting the operation

If you practice yoga regularly, you may already be aware of the subtle differences and similarities between the assorted styles of yoga. All types of yoga may help you cultivate mindfulness, heal your body, and promote overall health and wellness. Suppose you want to go deep into the process of awakening your Kundalini energy. In that case, it is advised that you use Kundalini yoga and meditation to interact with that energy and, ultimately, your spiritual nature.

CHAPTER 8: PSYCHIC INTUITION & KUNDALINI

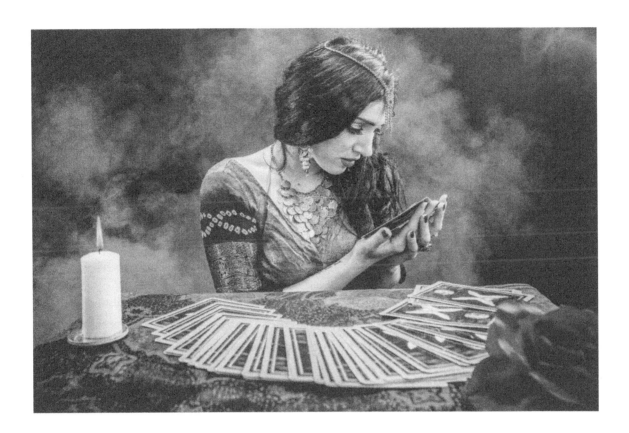

What Are Psychic Abilities?

Psychic abilities are considered supernatural abilities. Others might regard these skills to be impossible. However, it should be recognized that psychic powers are feasible and that people with such abilities exist. In reality, every human being possesses psychic powers. The issue is that most individuals do not hone their skills. As a result, they cannot employ and benefit from their powers. If individuals spent more time meditating, you'd notice that psychic powers are supposed to be pretty frequent. In reality, even simple breathing meditation practice daily might help you uncover your dormant psychic skills.

From now on, you should not regard psychic abilities as remarkable. Recognize that you have these abilities. It's simply a matter of honing and using your skills. Yes, you must learn how to use them efficiently.

Psychic powers have grown divisive. Some people do not believe in the existence of such powers at all. This is due to the unfortunate truth that many individuals who appear and claim to have psychic skills are simply scammers and hacks who do not even know how to meditate. Do not let these folks dissuade you from following a noble and magical path. The greatest way to confirm that such skills exist is to witness them yourself. The more you meditate, the more you will become aware of your psychic powers.

Different Psychic Abilities

The world is filled with people who have psychic talents. Although it would be ideal to master all of them, it would be more practical to focus your time and effort on mastering the one you enjoy the most. You can branch out and study another skill if you have extra time. Keep in mind that the quality of your learning must be prioritized. So, go ahead and study as many psychic talents as you like, but don't skimp on the quality of your education.

Numerous Psychic Ability Types

We'll go through the range of higher senses beyond the five physical senses. Consider that our five bodily senses are touch, smell, sight, hearing, and taste. They collaborate with the brain, a bodily organ, to gather information in the world outside of our physical realities to comprehend reality. However, we are more than our bodies. We are also spirit, emotion, and intellect, and it is only via these human qualities that we may reach greater levels of consciousness.

The conscious mind (awareness in everyday life), the subconscious mind (thoughts, feelings, information, and perceptions that lay below our conscious, waking mind), and the unconscious mind are the three accepted levels of consciousness (cognitive disconnection from the body, most commonly occurring in the deepest stages of sleep). Even if we aren't aware of it, these functions interact. We breathe without thinking, experience hunger when our bodies need food, are naturally compelled to use the restroom, and even have a desire for sexual connection. These natural activities stimulate our consciousness while we go about our everyday lives, executing the duties required of us to repeat our daily existence. Everything we do is recorded and stored by the subconscious. It detects our emotions and pushes us to respond. We are only dimly aware of the subtext of daily existence. However, by becoming aware of how our subconscious mind works, we may obtain a far more excellent knowledge of ourselves. Consider the power released, and you will instantly understand the significance.

The conscious mind is rational, analytical, observant, and organized in nature. The conscious mind's view is based on personal experience and acquired belief systems, and it can be altered by emotional involvement. In other words, no matter how bright we are, emotions and the limits of the conscious mind can cause us to make incorrect observations and conclusions. This reflects the distinction between knowledge and wisdom. Our conscious minds frequently tell us untrue information. To broaden our consciousness to cover the entirety of reality, we must engage our awareness in dialogue with the subconscious mind. That discussion provides an entry point to a more extended and developed awareness, capable of far more than our conscious mind is on its own.

The subconscious mind is a far more fertile ground than the conscious mind. It's bright, artistic, innovative, and symbolic. The subconscious is associated with dreams and assists us in making sense of our emotions and experiences. It is where our potential, understanding, consciousness, and innate powers (psychic and otherwise) may grow indefinitely. Great corporate leaders and innovators either have a natural ability or have taught themselves to function from the subconscious mind. It liberates individuals from the conscious mind's strict, structured approach to marketing, design, team management, and other areas. It also encourages an alternative, inspired intellectual approach that is both inventive and harmonious. Artists of many disciplines draw inspiration from the subconscious mind and its creative impulses.

The unconscious mind may appear inert, as though nothing happens there. It's difficult to imagine what it's doing, at least from a physical viewpoint, because our conscious minds cannot perceive its operation. All of the body's physiological functions (such as breathing and a heartbeat) are on autopilot, but any cognition associated with these activities is missing. The unconscious is more profound than the subconscious, which may be the source of imagination. This function of the mind is required to think of something higher than ourselves. We may connect with a tremendously coordinated and intricately connected living presence (the collective unconscious, in Jungian words) of which we are all a part. The unconscious is a portal to the collective unconscious through the subconscious mind that we all share.

Have you ever had a wonderful idea that might have led to implementing a plan, but you didn't take advantage of it? Maybe you'll see your concept put into action by someone else after some time. This represents the idea that we are all linked by a global unconscious network from which we may extract thoughts and process them into the physical world and that these ideas are available for us to find. If you don't act on an idea that occurs to you, someone else will, and it will become a reality.

So, what exactly are the various psychic abilities?

There are quite a few, but clairvoyance is one of the most well-known. Clairvoyance, often known as clear-seeing, is the capacity to perceive beyond what the naked eye can see. It can let you see beyond the present and divine the future and perceive and interpret auras and subtle energies and beings, among other things. Clairvoyance is linked to the Ajna chakra, the seat of intuition and higher awareness. If you wish to improve your psychic abilities, you must first strengthen your Ajna chakra.

Clairsentience, which translates as "clear feeling," is another term for the psychic ability you should be familiar with. It is the ability to receive intuitive signals through emotions and experiences, including bodily sensations. People that have this skill are known as empaths. This is related to their empathic abilities. This skill will allow you to feel and comprehend individuals on a much deeper level. This is distinguished by an increased sensitivity to subtle energies, moods, and emotions. The more you meditate, the more you will be able to develop this ability. This skill is more closely related to the heart chakra. Of course, the Ajna chakra plays a significant part in developing this psychic capacity.

Clear hearing is referred to as clairaudience. Consider it to be a small voice that instructs you what to do. You've heard the adage that there's an angel alongside you who occasionally guides you on what to do. It is often the psychic skill known as clairaudience that should be credited. Because it relies on intuition, this capacity is also related to the Ajna chakra. It's also worth noting that this psychic skill is frequently used to receive messages from the spiritual realm. Because individuals on the spiritual plane dwell in a distinct realm or plane of existence, you cannot expect them to manifest forcefully on the physical level.

Everyone has a good recall of having used this psychic skill. The "voice" speaks to you in your brain and tells you what to do or what to think about. Consider it to be communications from your guardian angel. Although we can get messages from our guardian angel, it is also true that some of these profound messages may originate from your intuition and be psychically relayed to you. The more you meditate, the more you will be able to recognize this "voice" in your brain. It's your instincts speaking to you. Pay attention to it.

Claircognizance, often known as clear understanding, is another intriguing psychic skill. It is the power to know things without recourse to reasoning or facts. You might think of it as a type of inner knowledge. For example, "knowing" that you should not trust a specific individual, only to discover that that person cannot be trusted or is a nasty person. Please keep in mind that this is different from clairaudience. You don't have to deal with any type of voice in this scenario. Instead, you simply know how things are. You are not required to do anything; you simply know. Although all of your chakras should be highly developed to master this power, two primary chakras are needed for this psychic ability: the crown chakra and the Ajna chakra.

So far, we've covered the most essential psychic skills. However, it should be emphasized that other additional psychic talents exist. Unfortunately, the world views the powers listed above as the "primary" abilities. The reality is that different skills are as impressive.

Telekinesis

Telekinesis is the psychic capacity to move items with one's thoughts. This is one of the most intriguing skills you can master. It is also quite well-liked. But the issue remains: Is it true? Yes. Learning telekinesis, on the other hand, takes time and practice. If you wish to study telekinesis, here are the steps you need to take:

Place a light item, preferably on a table, in front of you. You may use a feather, a little stone, or anything lightweight. Now sit back and relax. Concentrate on the item in front of you. Create a tunnel between yourself and the thing. Nothing should be in front of you but the object of your attention. Visualize your astral hand reaching out and pushing the thing away from you. Another thing you may do is imagine a Prana ray pushing the item. Keep an eye on it.

As you can see, the steps are straightforward. It is up to you to practice this method until you are proficient at it. Once you've mastered it, you may skip the portion where you have to imagine a tunnel between yourself and the thing. Its sole goal is to assist you in visualizing and focusing.

Another Method to Perform Telekinesis

Put something in front of you. Simply unwind. Concentrate on the object now. Try to feel it. Be a part of it. Think of the item as an extension of yourself. What is it like to be the object? Do you have a sense of how it (you) is related to the table? Be a part of it. The more you become one with it, the more you will feel as if you can move it, similar to how you would move your hand. When you eventually get to the point where you are one with the thing — that you are the object — simply move, and it will carry with you.

It is critical to become one with the thing to the point that you believe it has become a part of you. Another thing to remember is to avoid using force. You must be calm when practicing telekinesis. When concentrating on something, it is usual to utilize force. Keep in mind that concentration does not necessitate the application of force. The less stressed you are, the better. The most crucial factor is your mental condition.

Telekinesis is classified into two types: micro kinesis and macro kinesis. The two procedures described above are instances of macro kinesis, which is the movement of things. If you believe it will be too tough for you, you might begin with micro kinesis. Micro kinesis deals with unpredictability instead of physically manipulating items with your thoughts. Here's an activity you may try to practice micro kinesis.

Use a random number generator. If you like, you may use a dice or a coin. The goal of micro kinesis is to influence the result of randomness. Instead of moving an object, you should produce a specific outcome. For example, flip a coin and ensure that the head side is facing up. You may also shuffle a deck of cards and use your ability to ensure that the top card is always red. Again, micro kinesis is about affecting the outcome of chance. So, how do you go about doing this? It is analogous to moving an object. Let us use a die for this practice. The goal is to have it land on the number 6 (the number 6 facing up). The procedure is as follows:

Hold the die in your hand and relax. Before you roll it, imagine that the outcome is number 6. Visualize this in your thoughts several times. Be one with the dice by feeling it in your palm. You will get the impression that you are one with the die and can control it to roll whatever number you desire. Now, roll the dice confidently, knowing that the result will be the number of your choosing. It is number 6 in this situation. You can also try another number.

You are allowed to create your approach or workout. The premise stays the same: You should see the item and become one with it. Never, ever, ever employ any type of force. Remember that you do not push things to happen; instead, you just allow them to happen.

The Hundredth Monkey Theory

This theory is said to have emerged in Japan in 1952 due to research on Macaque monkeys. Lyall Watson detailed the study and its conclusions in an introduction to Lawrence Blair's book *Rhythms of Vision*, released in 1975. It was determined, in essence, that taught habits reach a "tipping point" at which these behaviors or abilities spread exponentially throughout an identifiable group and peripheral groups, effectively normalizing them. That behavior was washing sweet potatoes in the case of the monkeys observed. The talents were passed on generationally and subsequently socially to surrounding groups by the monkeys. The notion gained popularity because of Ken Keyes Jr.'s book *The 100th Monkey.*

The theory is founded on the concept that once a clever idea, habit, or talent achieves a specific degree of widespread saturation (the 100th monkey), its spread will be accelerated until it becomes normative. While it does not match the theoretical pattern of the 100th monkey, it does imply something quite similar - that ideas and behaviors reach a point where they are unavoidably accepted internationally. The same conceptual framework may describe the spread of higher consciousness as an attainable and desirable objective for all humans.

While the scientific community continues to argue against this impact, it is evident that ideas frequently reach certain levels of public consciousness, causing them to spread in all directions and become internationally accepted. This is demonstrably true. Malcolm Gladwell's book *The Tipping Point: How Little Things Can Make a Big Difference* is a re-imagining of the 100th monkey idea, which is applied to the effect seen in the dissemination of trends and goods. It's undeniable that the hypothesis has a lot of truth to it. Furthermore, the same idea may be used to diffusion higher consciousness and the human knowledge of our communal intimacy in the collective unconscious network.

Have you ever considered how advertisements influence your perception of things? You may not be aware of it, but your subconscious mind is constantly being given information, which may be altering the way you think. You must be able to realize that your degree of consciousness — or awareness — will constantly be influenced by stimuli around you.

With the help of modern technology such as the Internet, we may be approaching that tipping point. This signifies a significant evolutionary transition in human development. Intuition is far more powerful than you may realize. If you learn to harness it, you will discover that you can read people much more effectively — not allowing preconceived notions to come in the way of authentic assessment.

The strength of intuition has been researched by scientists for ages and has even been utilized to deter criminal activity. You might be interested in reading research that indicates a pattern behind what occurs to a human being depending on their conduct and reaction to others. We learn to react as a group, which isn't necessarily the ideal response. Just as the 100th monkey idea may be used to acquire beautiful outcomes; it can also generate disastrous consequences if we set instinct aside and disregard it. The signs and signals are all around us, yet we choose to ignore them. In his book *The Gift of Fear*, Gavin De Becker utilized our lack of intuitive reaction to explain how humans ignore their instincts and place themselves in circumstances that are not just unpredictable but hazardous.

On the other hand, psychics can pick up on messages from their intuition and are not fearful of what those signals are saying. It's fascinating reading, and it could even explain to readers why intuition is so vital to trust. Psychics worth their salt will recognize that the inner knowing that contemporary dogma may choke is always present if you can peel away all the taught resistance to follow that inner wisdom. Advertisements on television may instill preconceived notions about what is good and evil, whereas the intuitive nature of the psychic will look past this.

The Unconscious and Dreams

Simply recalling dreams is an example of bringing information from the subconscious into consciousness. Dreams are the result of our unconscious thoughts. There are several ideas on the purpose of dreams. While each has merit, many dream researchers who base their thinking on the work of famed psychologist Carl Jung feel that dreams are a safe area to symbolically act out emotions and scenarios of concern from our waking lives. According to this notion, Dreams help us resolve the emotional outflow and worry that might occur from stress and the more unpleasant parts of life without causing unnecessary damage.

From the standpoint of the brain, the deepest sleep stage places us in the domain of the unconscious. The only measurable brainwave activity in this state is the delta wave, which is incredibly slow and one of four known to exist in our various states of awareness. Subconscious brain waves are largely theta (the slowest kind after delta) waves, observed in yogis and Buddhist monks after entering profound stages of meditation, as well as alpha waves, prevalent during dream states. Beta waves are the quickest brainwaves, and they are most prevalent during being awake. These waves help us organize, prioritize, and manage activities in our daily lives and those requiring fine motor or cognitive skills. The length of a wave dictates the nature of the substance and the radiation it produces, which is inversely proportional to its frequency. Are you starting to see a pattern here?

EQ

These letters stand for "emotional quotient," which reflects our capacity to detect the emotional states of others and ourselves and the general emotional condition of a room full of people. People with a high EQ are also known as "empaths" because they are particularly emotionally sensitive for a good reason. Emotions continually influence people, and how we choose to cope with those emotions affects our entire physical and mental health. Emotions are inescapable, and while our environment impacts relationships, events, and locations, they are entirely under our control.

Those with high EQs may perceive the mental state of others better than others. Furthermore, they are acutely aware of things such as subtext (both in terms of what isn't conveyed with words and the emotional context of the words themselves). This is the substance that diplomats and mindful medicine are made of and those in all therapeutic professions. It's what teachers, politicians, and clever leaders of all types rely on to follow the professions in which they were created to use their skills. High EQ persons can dig more deeply into the reality of such encounters, evaluating their genuine substance, rather than using the complex experiences, prejudices, and societal assumptions that most people use in their relationships with others. People with a high level of emotional intelligence can hear beyond words and see past the surface of things to get to the heart of the matter. They understand that there is always more behind the hood and aren't afraid to use that knowledge to find solutions that respect the individuals involved. They know that one size does not fit everyone. They also realize that reluctance might encourage them to ask questions or recognize that there is more to learn.

Even if someone looks emotionless, they may have established the practice of suppressing their emotions to disguise them. Emotions, on the other hand, do not go away. They are kept in the body and, if not properly released, will remain there, building up like air pressure in a small container. Repressed emotions can cause obstructions in our bodies' energy pathways. When these blockages build, our physical and mental health suffers because everything inside us isn't flowing as it should. As a result, empaths must find appropriate outlets for their feelings.

Have you ever gone into a room where two people had recently argued and felt the tension in the air without saying anything? If so, you were picking up on the emotional vibrations that the dispute emitted in the room. This is an example of a psychic reaction. Nobody is required to say anything to you. They don't have to show you their behavior, but you can sense their emotional condition. Your higher senses detect the emotional vibrations conveyed by other people's emotional states, which have a lingering influence on the environment.

It can be challenging for empaths to work fluidly throughout their lives without understanding what is going on and knowing how to guard themselves against being pulled one way or another every time they encounter an emotional vibrational field. Each emotion has its frequency. Negative emotions have a lower frequency, and happy emotions have a greater frequency. Often, empaths will feel emotional and have no idea why, assuming that these feelings are being created by them and attempting to find out why they are feeling that way. It may be highly unsettling, but the empath's capacity to detect other people's emotional states, when properly recognized, can also be a gift.

Telepathy

Telepathy is the capacity to perceive what others are thinking (also described as minding reading). Twins, close pals, and emotionally attached lovers are examples of people who can read each other's minds and often finish each other's sentences without looking at each other. So, do they have psychic abilities, or do they just know each other so well that they can predict where their stream of thought would go in any situation? In this debate, the expression "being on the same page" comes to mind, which might be adapted to "being on the same frequency level" with your growing understanding of how the universe works.

This skill comes in a variety of forms. While some people think they are psychic, they are not. Some people are simply gifted at reading others, and there are training schools available worldwide to educate people on how to do so. It's an issue of knowing what posture and body postures say about people's emotional and psychological states. We pick up on and react to many signals conveyed by people's body language and speech patterns without even recognizing them. It's the result of one subconscious connecting with another.

Listening is another ability that increases your awareness. Develop your listening skills so that you are not just hearing what someone is saying and are not assuming anything but can determine what they genuinely mean from their words. This interprets the "subtext" (meaning behind the meaning) of what is expressed with words. This is a crucial talent since it helps you read between the lines and grasp what people aren't saying.

True telepathy is having such a clean mind that you are devoid of thinking and receptive to absorbing information through the Third Eye-opening. It may feel ridiculous and nonsensical at first, and you must trust the process. This skill allows you to receive communications that may seem random and unimportant to you.

However, with time and effort, you will discover that messages and information obtained through an open Third Eye apply to individuals around you. You'll quickly be able to locate significance in them if you strengthen your intuitive abilities.

Pyrokinesis

Another psychic skill that will allow you to control fire is pyrokinesis. Many individuals would be interested in learning this approach. Pyrokinesis requires practice to master like any other kinetic skill, but it is well worth it. You will need a candle for this exercise. The procedure is as follows:

Light the candle. Relax. Concentrate your attention now on the candle's flame. Be a part of it. It's palpable. Consider yourself to be the flame. Do you have a sense of how hot you are? This flame is a manifestation of oneself. Spend some more time getting to know the flame. Once you've reached this stage of oneness with the flame, you'll be able to feel as if you can move it. Allow it to tilt to one side, then the other. Keep in mind that you are the flame.

You might also use visualization to shift the candle flame. If you entirely become one with the flame, you will not need to put in too much effort. It's as if you can feel it and want it to move. The same ideas apply here — merging with the item and visualization. You might not even need to employ visualization if you get skilled at it. This is determined by your spiritual growth as well as your personal preferences. The best approach to finding out what will work for you is to experiment and discover what works.

Other additional psychic skills might be addressed. However, to accomplish them, another book, or several volumes, would be required to cover everything. You have all of the knowledge you need to activate and strengthen your psychic senses for the time being. Let us now move on to the topic of psychic awareness.

Psychic Perception

Psychic awareness is not a psychic skill in and of itself, but it is the proper strategy to adopt while awakening your psychic senses. "With great power comes tremendous responsibility," as the adage goes. You might think your psychic abilities are unusual if you're just starting. This is because you haven't gotten acclimated to them yet. However, the more you practice the meditation techniques in this book, the more in touch you will be with your psychic senses. They will soon become prevalent and typical for you. Because meditation activates all of the chakras, you may be sure that if you follow the techniques in this book rigorously, you will develop various psychic senses/abilities.

It is critical to be aware of the existence of energy and the quality of this energy when it comes to being attentive. For example, if you meet someone and detect a strong negative vibe from them, you may want to avoid them or, at the very least, put up a shield when speaking with them. You may use your psychic senses to benefit you in your daily life if you are psychically aware.

You should realize that if you don't employ your psychic senses, they won't be able to aid you.

It's worth noting that the term "psychic" is derived from the word psi, which means "energy." As a result, when you talk about psychic awareness, you're talking about being aware of the energy inside you and all around you. By detecting and comprehending energy, you will be better equipped to choose the right course of action in every scenario. As a result, it can assist you in making the best decision and plan of action.

Empathy

Another psychic skill that will allow you to detect human emotions and moods is empathy. Empathy is the key to developing psychic awareness. Technically, you can catch more than simple emotions when you gain empathy. Instead, you learn to see and comprehend energy, particularly the quality of energy.

So, how do you cultivate empathy? Again, the activities in this book might help you build empathy. You may also engage in specific techniques to improve this skill directly. Let us go over them one by one:

Empathic Bonding

The next time you engage with someone, imagine a cord connecting your heart chakra to the other person's heart chakra. Maintain a clear and open mind. What are your thoughts about it? Is there anything that comes to mind when you connect with this person? Try to detect the other person's state of mind. When you're finished, don't forget to sever the connection. You can do this by psychically imagining yourself severing the bond with a pair of scissors or a knife.

Psychic Perception

Simply being motionless and feeling the other person is a straightforward approach to developing empathy. What are your thoughts about them? You must clear your thoughts before using this technique. Having a clear mind will help you pick up on the other person's perceptions. To learn more about and comprehend the other person, use your intuition and psychic senses.

Empowering the Heart Chakra

The heart chakra is the primary chakra for empathy. As a result, you can be more sympathetic by growing your heart chakra. There is a simple but efficient approach to achieve this: Charge your heart chakra with energy. Imagine that you are drawing energy from the cosmos and allowing it to flow and charge up your heart chakra every time you inhale. Allow the heart chakra to be activated until it appears brightly in your mind's eye. Do this numerous times a day, and you will undoubtedly have a powerful heart chakra that you can utilize to empathize with others successfully.

Pay Attention to Your Emotions/Feelings

Empathy is all about feelings or emotions. The more you learn the language of sensations, the more you will be able to understand what certain energy impressions signify. As a result, make it a practice to train yourself to listen to your emotions. The better you comprehend particular emotions, the more you will grasp the language accompanying them.

Some people only get in touch with their psychic powers or senses when they meditate or conduct something relevant to their spiritual practice. This is incorrect since you cannot truly separate your psychic self from who you are, even during normal consciousness. As a result, you must learn to live with your psychic powers and perceptions.

Astral Travel

Another fascinating topic is astral travel or astral projection. It is thought that when a person sleeps, their astral body splits from their physical body and travels to the astral realm. However, the difficulty is that most people do not remember what happened during their astral excursions. Yes, astral projection occurs naturally. You must, however, learn to be mindful and recall your trip. This is why you should deliberately practice astral projection. It's also worth noting that meditation can assist you in learning astral travel.

Inducing Astral Projection

The Technique of Implementation

This is a widespread and successful method of astral projection. The goal here is to go into a profound meditation before rolling out. Rather than rolling with your physical body, your astral body will roll out and split from your physical body. You must identify as the astral body rather than the physical body. "You have a body, but the body is not you," as the phrase goes. The procedure is as follows:

To guarantee the free passage of energy, lie down and make sure your spine is straight. Relax. Feel yourself sinking further and deeper into a trance with each inhalation. Feel the astral body trapped in a physical body, not the gross physical body. Be more in touch with your astral body. Allow your body to sleep while being aware. When you notice your body has fallen asleep, imagine yourself as the astral body and roll to the side.

If you complete the task correctly, you will be able to roll out with your astral body. Don't be startled if you become detached and see your actual body lying on the bed.

Flying

If you experience dreams where you are flying, it is a good indication that you were on an astral journey. This is one of the most effective methods to do it on purpose. It is possible to achieve full-fledged astral travel by inducing the state of being able to fly. The procedure is as follows:

Maintain a straight spine by lying down comfortably. Relax. Visualize your astral body gradually emerging from your physical body. Associate with and identify with this astral body. Look down and notice how blissfully your physical body is resting. You have entered the astral dimension. Allow yourself to float to the ceiling. How does your room appear? Now, hover higher above your house and see your surroundings. Take in the beautiful environment around you. Feel the frigid wind brush up against your astral body. Raise your head farther higher towards the sky. Keep an eye on the stars and the moon. Fly about and see various places and individuals. On this voyage, you may encounter some astral entities; for the time being, disregard them. Continue to fly around the Earth and explore it. Allow yourself to go more into this condition. If done correctly, this simple mental exercise can lead to a full-fledged astral excursion. Simply think about your actual body and will yourself back to it if you desire to return to it. "I am back in my physical body," you say as you move your fingers and toes. Open your eyes slowly and recite a short prayer.

It should be emphasized that some astral travelers report returning to their physical body with a headache, which can be slight or severe. This is usually due to the effect, especially if you travel to a distant location. As a result, it is advised that you do not return to your physical body right away. Instead, simply return to your room and see your physical body lying on the bed; only once in your room should you enter your physical body.

Will

An act of will can also be used to cause astral travel. Simply will yourself out of your body if you are already in a profound trance. If you know you have strong willpower, this is a fantastic strategy to apply. You should also utilize your visualizing abilities to make it more effective.

Feel your astral body separate from your physical body. Take notice that you must first enter a trance state before attempting an astral project. Be careful not to become overly connected to your physical body. Recognize that you are an astral creature who only inhabits a physical body.

Is It Dangerous?

When people talk about astral travel, one of the first questions they ask is if it is harmful. Can you get hurt, or worse, die, while you astral travel? There are, of course, opposing viewpoints on this subject. However, the vast majority of people believe that astral travel is risk-free.

Consider this: Every night while you sleep, you are already astral traveling (just like everyone else). You've done it hundreds of times. It is just a matter of being aware and in command of this behavior.

If you're still concerned about your safety, here are some precautions you may take to guarantee a safe astral journey:

- Keep a glass of saltwater nearby. A glass of saltwater is thought to repel bad energy and beings.
- Visualize a bubble of safety surrounding your body before you astral project, shielding you from all harm.
- Place something alongside you. Wear it instead, if feasible.
- Before making an astral projection, apply saltwater to your body.
- Before attempting astral projection, pray for protection and guidance.

- Request assistance from the angels or your guardian angel. Your guardian angel is said to be able to hear you at any time.

Astral projection may be entertaining. However, it takes time and practice to master, much like any other skill. It's also worth noting that while you astral travel, you may quickly be yanked back to your physical body if you feel too much excitement or terror. This is why you must remain as calm as possible throughout. When individuals see their bodies lying on the bed, they are usually jerked back to their actual selves. This is primarily related to anxiety. All you have to do is get used to it. Remember that fear will bring you back to your body if you are on a journey, which is another reason why astral traveling is incredibly safe. When you perceive danger, your attention is drawn back to your body. You may also return to your physical body just by willpower.

A prevalent issue nowadays is a lack of practice. If you have a lot on your plate, you might wish to practice astral projection every night before bed or when you wake up. It is also not recommended to do astral projects if you are already exhausted, as you will fall asleep. In this situation, you could wish to try astral projection first thing in the morning.

Astral travel is a fascinating skill to acquire. When you learn how to astral travel, you will be able to experience many great experiences and teachings.

CHAPTER 9: ASCENSION OF THE MIND, CONSCIOUSNESS, AND TRANSCENDENCE

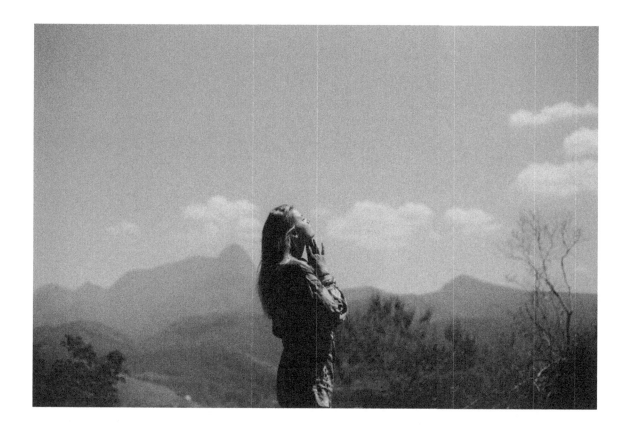

Energy is an alive and tactile life force that we can all grasp in the context of our daily lives. We frequently blame poor energy levels on a lousy diet, a lack of sleep, or even the weather. The most crucial problem, though, is more convoluted than it appears. Our energy systems may be damaged by emotional, physical, and even cognitive obstacles that we have accumulated from childhood and are unaware of.

Consciousness and Energy

The word is frequently molded into scientific or even mystical definitions. In attempting to describe it, we lose sight of the worth or more profound knowledge of energy.

Everything we know about energy is that we should be calm, relax ourselves, and be aware of our surroundings. For example, when we feel present, our energy is anchored, and when we experience repulsion or attraction, our energy is charged. When we laugh or weep, we feel the energy leave our bodies. Certain events, and yes, individuals, may sap our energy, as can certain locales. On the other hand, we cling to people, events, and places that feed our energy source when we feel insufficient.

Energy cannot be generated or destroyed, but it may be manipulated. We can accelerate or decelerate energy, and it can exist in closed systems where it can aid, or it can exist in an open system where energy flows. Uncontained energy might generate a fractured or frenzied system. Similarly, depleting energy can lead to the collapse of a system.

Despite its strength, energy is a neutral force. It is a consciousness that controls its movement. When we view energy in the same way we see awareness, we become more direct in our energy's movement toward connection, creativity, and evolution. The less aware you are, the more energy separates you from others.

Energy Blockage

Our minds are open and flexible, and our breathing is regular and deep, creating a sense of spaciousness in our bodies. We can achieve a healthy balance of constriction and expansion and activation and receptivity in Kundalini flow.

We allow our thinking, emotions, and will to collaborate. In the process, we develop faith in ourselves and, at times, discover ourselves undefended- this is referred to as energy integrity. Energy integrity is fleeting, and many individuals describe it as static, obstructed, or even trapped. This is a minimal way of thinking since their respiration and posture are not addressed.

Helpful Hints for Understanding Your Energy System

1. Because our ideas are also kinds of energy, we must become conscious of what we are thinking. One of the first things you may do is start your day by thinking about your first thought of the day and then proceed from there. You may even construct a list of things to do. Just take note of the words you use and how they make you feel.

2. Try to give yourself a break throughout the day by pausing whatever you're doing, closing your eyes, and going within to feel where you are. What do you feel at the moment? How does your breathing feel? Are you keeping it a secret? How do you feel in your body — relaxed or tense? Restricted? Tired? Alive?

3. Pay attention to your energy even when you're moving. Move your body, moving different portions at a time, and notice how you feel as you do so. Do you have any ideas or sensations that come to mind? Is there a certain portion of your body that becomes electrified when you move? Is there anything that has piqued your interest? Do you feel the urge to keep your energies under check?

4. Make noises by yourself or with others. The goal here is to let your voice be heard. What are your thoughts? Are you feeling energized? Take note of how you feel when you say YES or NO. Which one is easier to express? Are you willing to repeat that noise or sound? Take note of all of these details without passing judgment.

5. Pay attention to what happens to your energy when you are in the company of others and how your body feels around them and how your breathing changes—does it expand or contract?

6. Don't be hesitant to experiment with your boundaries. You can use a companion to accompany you in this active boundary exploring. Simply stand a distance apart and, as you move closer to each other simultaneously, discover how you sense their energy. Make mental notes about what occurs to you when another person's energy enters your energy field. Do you have a sense of being more or less grounded? Do you feel in command or as though you're losing yourself? Do you believe you have the ability to speak up?

7. Take notes on your various feelings — what are your associations with these sensations, and what pictures or thoughts come to mind when these feelings arise? How and where do you address these emotions?

8. How and where do you feel most at ease meeting the rest of the world? Many of us say this at home, but think about the circumstances and locations you've been in, and are you comfortable with yourself? How do you lead using emotions, logic, and willpower? How do you feel about the other if you do lead with one? What portions of your body do you utilize to interact with the outside world? Do you solely utilize your brain, heart, or hands, or do you use a combination of all three?

9. Seek out someone else's experience with your energy and see how they connect to it — how do you feel in their presence, and how do they feel in yours? Are you invited and at ease, or are you uninvited and held at bay? Is there a separation? Do you have the impression that they are withholding something? Do you want to collapse?

This list may appear lengthy, but the truth is that we experience a wide range of emotions when we are confronted with situations, objects, or people. The questions above simply help us become more aware and point to what we can look out for to pin down our feelings and try to understand them. It assists us in studying how we act and respond, and it improves our ability to sense our energy and the energies of those around us.

Detecting Energy

Sensing energy is the hardest thing to perform immediately out of all the things you may do. This is not a regular occurrence. However, there are strategies for sensing and manipulating energy that you may use:

1. As with anything else, close your eyes and begin by envisioning your entire body, including all of its veins.

2. Imagine the veins you see, but instead of imagining them red with blood, imagine them transporting energy, which may be any color you associate with. Observe the electricity around your body, contacting every neuron.

3. Next, try noticing the vibrations when this energy passes throughout your body.

4. Concentrate on a particular body part, such as the arms, and direct the energy in your body to that location. If you feel or detect any tingling sensations, it is most likely the result of successful energy manipulation. Repeat with your other arm before moving on to your legs.

5. Once you've finished transferring the energy throughout your body, let it flow freely back through your body.

Don't be disheartened if you don't feel anything the first time or even a few times afterward. Energy manipulation is complex; thus, it requires experience, patience, and time.

Programming

Programming is the most important aspect of energy manipulation. There are several methods to program, and various approaches work better for different people.

Chakras and Energy Manipulation

Chakras may or may not be beneficial or even required in energy manipulation. Still, it is always crucial to check your chakra balance and ensure they are not clogged because energy runs via chakras. If your chakras are blocked, you may not be able to manipulate energy.

Absorbing Energy

There are several methods for absorbing energy. It might come from outside sources, but it could also come from within us. Chakras can also be immersed in circumstances, locations, and experiences.

Here's what you can do if you wish to absorb energy:

1. Select a target from which you wish to absorb energy. It is beneficial to obtain energy from inanimate objects such as trees or flowers. This source of energy must not interfere with the energy you are receiving.
2. Concentrate on the thing, and then connect yourself and the object. You may make this easier by imagining a cable linking you and this thing.
3. Visualize the passage of energy from the thing to you. Take only what you require and nothing more.

If you intend to absorb energy from another individual, you must always obtain their permission first. Not asking for permission may result in negative outcomes because the energy was gained accidentally or without authorization.

You can also absorb energy from your surroundings. This is known as ambient energy, and retrieving it is as simple as visualizing a connection to the energy from where you are standing or sitting.

Releasing energy is frequently done only when you've taken too much of it. All you have to do is reverse the steps outlined above.

Activate Transcendence

Consider yourself a conduit for energy to enter and fill your body. As an energy receiver, you must set aside your anxieties, ego, and thoughts. Consider yourself to be a hollow capsule. You are an open doorway through which the energy of the cosmos can flow. If you begin each meditation with these ideas, you will find it simpler to achieve a soothing, serene condition.

When you enter your sacred space, leave your earthly problems at the door. You are no longer on this planet. You're ascending to a greater level of consciousness. This should be done whether you are practicing alone or doing a reading for someone else. You will discover powerful psychic skills to help you achieve any objective you set for yourself. Whether it's reading one's emotions, seeing another location on Earth or in the cosmos, getting communications from another planet or time, or discovering a lost thing, it starts with a centering meditation.

Psychometry

Psychometry was invented in 1842 and has been used for centuries. It refers to the capacity to read a thing via touch. The thing has a history that may be read by someone focused and receptive to energy. A psychic will concentrate and establish a channel for energy to enter. The psychic will either hold the thing in their hands or set it before them. They are hoping for particular feelings or visuals to emerge. They may occasionally sense what the person was like, what they did, and how they died. It is up to the psychic to tell the individual what they want them to know while remaining cautious only to express what they know to be true. No matter how competent the psychic is, they may not always be able to interpret all objects.

These talents, such as holding an object or being in the same room as someone, may be straightforward. The quantity of mental energy and focus necessary, on the other hand, is never simple. It is critical to remember to remain motionless and empty at all times. If your mind wanders, you may have to close the door and restart. Keep the meditation going for as long as you need to feel ready to accept energy.

Automatic Writing

You can take as much time as you need to center yourself. Prepare a pen and paper or a computer, whichever method you want. Fill in the blanks with whatever comes to mind. Your conscious ideas will soon fade into the background, and subconscious thoughts will flow from your fingertips. Continue writing for as long as you like or as long as your thoughts last. Many psychics who utilize this approach are unaware of what they have written until they read it.

Doodling is a type of instinctive writing since it is not actively targeted. The spiral, related to sacred geometry, is one of the most prevalent doodles. It is advised that if you have emotional issues, you should avoid attempting to write automatically. You are more likely to attract a lower-frequency entity since your frequency is lower because of emotional problems. Similarly, if you are surrounded by continual turmoil in your life, you should avoid attempting to channel it. To assist you in writing, it is necessary to adjust your emphasis, moving your brain from left-brain logical to right-brain intuitive. Pretend you're getting ready to write; put pen to paper, then move on to something else. The majority of individuals will write something coherent. Messages may be written in a foreign language or an unfamiliar writing style and signed by someone else.

You'll figure out who's writing through you if you're at ease. Stop if you feel even the slightest bit uneasy about the information you're receiving or the entity writing through you. If more than one entity is attempting to write via you, politely request that they be patient and allow you to address them one at a time. Make a note of the name.

Channeling

Receiving sights, sounds, or sensations from another realm is all about channeling. The capacity to receive communications from a higher entity or realm is known as clairaudience. The psychic can hear numerous sounds, such as whispers or a clear, booming voice, even though no one else is in the room. Clairsentience, a psychic empath, is the capacity to read emotions. Those who have this capacity can detect others' sentiments, powerful emotions, wrath, hostility, or symptoms of stress. They are skilled at reading body language. The empath can interpret the atmosphere regardless of whether they are at work, the grocery store, a party, or simply at home. They can read other people's emotions and know how they are feeling.

Finally, clairvoyance, often known as clear vision, is the capacity to view pictures from other levels of existence. Folks with clairvoyance can look into the future, the past, and the present. The Third Eye controls this talent. Concentrating on this chakra will assist in improving the visuals. The visuals may be crisp and in focus or hazy and foggy.

Dowsing

Dowsing uses hand-held equipment to search for information or anything concealed from view. Dowsing developed as a method of locating subsurface water, which is not unexpected given that water is a requirement for humans. Many people are unaware that it may also be used to find metals or ores, jewels, oil, gravesites, and occasionally missing individuals. Dowsing is a skill anybody can learn if they have the proper training and instruments. Like many other psychic skills, children have an inherent talent for dowsing. The instruments employed are an extension of a person's innate talent, allowing them to notice things they would not have been able to discover otherwise. Dowsing tools include the following:

- **V Rod:** Originally fashioned of forked twigs, a V rod can today be manufactured of any springy material, such as wood, cane, plastic, or metal. When it detects something, the V rod will jerk upward.
- **Angel Rods:** Angel rods are two L-shaped rods, with the dowser holding the rod by the short arm and the extended part parallel to the ground. The lengthier parts will cross when the dowser discovers anything underground.

- **Wand:** A wand is a long rod held in one's hand and travels in circular or oscillating motions when it senses anything.
- **Pendulum:** A pendulum is often a crystal strung with twine to a rod that allows it to swing freely. It can react to varied motions and is typically used for distant dowsing using charts or maps.

Extrasensory Perception (ESP)

ESP is a type of intuition. At all times, the psychic can see energy bouncing off the universe. This capacity, like breathing, feels natural. There are several levels of intuition. An intuitive can give guidance based on their ability to interpret energy in their surroundings. A medical intuitive is a psychic who can read bodies, either their own or others, to diagnose pain, disease, or injury. They tune into health issues and use therapeutic massage, reiki, acupressure, or acupuncture to heal. A psychic detective is someone who can discern energy at crime scenes. ESP is a catch-all phrase for psychic abilities such as telepathy, clairvoyance, precognition, and clairaudience.

J.B. Rhine and his wife, Louisa E. Rhine, explored ESP for the first time at Duke University in the 1930s. J.B. worked in the lab, developing the term ESP and creating techniques to test it, while Louise mostly collected experiences of ESP. He made Zener cards, including the symbols circle, square, wavy lines, cross, and star. A deck of 25 cards had five cards with each symbol. J.B. would put a psychic's clairvoyance to the test by concealing the cards while the psychic tried to predict the sequence.

Medium

A medium is a psychic who can converse with spirits by opening their mind and body. When a human body dies, the energy it contains must be released someplace. Many people think it is where spirits originate. These psychics can communicate with creatures who have gone on and have a message for loved ones. Most people who work in this sector are born with this skill and are aware of its potency from an early age. Voices and sentiments come quickly to them. Mediums usually only channel those who have just died, rather than people who have been dead for decades. The Ouija board is a popular kind of mediumship that anybody may use. Mediums may utilize knocking, rapping, or bell ringing to communicate with the departed. Mediums will also go into a trance to perform séances and sometimes channel spirits.

Readers

Psychic readers are those who conduct readings using instruments. They may employ any combination of leaves, runes, tarot cards, astrological charts, and numerology charts. Readers employ cartomancy, tarot, or divination cards to inform people of potential obstacles that may prevent them from realizing their full potential. Readers frequently perform palm readings. The lines, wrinkles, contours, and curves of the palm predict someone's future. This form of reading necessitates psychic abilities.

Scrying

The psychic sees pictures in water or on bright surfaces. Mirrors or two-way mirrors can also be used. The visuals give information that the psychic may utilize to assist the person using their services. Scrying is not a distinct psychic skill. The psychic's personal preferences determine how it is carried out. Nostradamus, a French apothecary and psychic, used scrying to predict the future by peering into a water bowl.

Telepathy

This is similar to being a psychic empath. It is not a matter of interpreting someone's feelings. The psychic can read people's minds and get information without communicating. Many psychics who have this ability can read the minds of every person they encounter. Only sometimes are they unable to penetrate people's thoughts.

Here's a fun technique to see if you're psychic:

Request that a buddy (the one you can rely on not to make fun of you) sit in a different room with playing cards. Turn each card over one at a time, striking a bell as they do so. Your companion must mentally describe the card to you. Write down what you believe the card is once you hear the bell. Compare your list to the real order of the cards once you've gone through the deck. If you get less than 20 correct, your psychic ability is limited. You have moderate psychic ability if you score between 20 and 30. If you get a score of 30 or higher, you are entirely psychic.

The Trance Channel

This is the pinnacle of employing oneself as a psychic power instrument. This power necessitates the psychic leaving their body and allowing someone else to enter. The psychic will be in a trance and talk in a different voice. They will be speaking in the other person's voice. This level of psychic talent is quite advanced. It requires a lot of focus and practice. Psychics can communicate with spirit guides or entities. Because they lack a physical embodiment, most are entities. Channels can access highly advanced creatures, which means they can contact people who have been missing for decades.

There are several methods to put your gifts to use, all of which begin with a meditation to concentrate your mind. Meditation is incredibly beneficial. It will be tough to develop advanced skills without first learning meditation.

Ascension

The ascension of the mind represents humanity's elevation to a greater degree of intellectual strength, in which the link we all share through the collective unconscious is more wholly recognized. All good must originate within you, and this is the primary notion of keeping in mind when you engage in contemplative practice. It's not all about you, my friend. It's all about us. It just flows from you initially, as it must from each individual.

On the opposite side of the planet, a butterfly flaps its wings, and the vibrations of that flap are felt across the world. Your thoughts and your capacity to master them start a universal consciousness process that dramatically influences the integrity of that consciousness by enhancing its quality. Consider what would happen if we all did this. Imagine if we could all spread our wings simultaneously and be felt in our vast numbers and boundless strength.

You'll know you're getting signals from your subconscious mind when they seem correct. You will have no question because they will approach you with conviction. You may not grasp all that is offered right now, but you will in time. Once you've mastered the capacity to settle your conscious mind into stillness, you may practice growing your psychic talents by imagining a question, asking it, then releasing it and returning to the silence. Depending on the inquiry, you will receive an answer, a message from your mind, or the universal unconscious. Experiment with different questions, even those you may learn the solution to later, with verifiable results. You could wish to inquire about who will be the next president or when a cure for cancer will be discovered. Look for questions with reliable answers. This is a solid approach to guarantee you're not delusory and that you're genuinely succeeding by developing the power to draw forth the treasures of your subconscious and what lies beyond it: the collective unconscious.

Because this is not an exact science, which may explain why it is not empirically established, the answers you receive at first may be muted, imprecise, or otherwise erroneous compared to how the answers play out in life. Some questions are not supposed to have answers. Sometimes we need to have a life experience to comprehend the consequences completely. However, keep in mind that the more you practice, the clearer and more precise your abilities will become.

Finally, meditation practice is a gift to yourself, the planet, and the people around you. You may become a source of peace for others by being more fully grounded in the truth of who you are and what your purpose in the world is. The serenity and tranquility you seek via contemplative practice have a rippling effect like that faraway butterfly. It spreads outward in concentric rings, touching people in their zone of influence. As these circles expand, so does their power to lure others into their orbit. The peaceful core you've discovered is shared reality. It's not only there to make you feel better, stronger, or "better." It exists to shift the mountains of despair that crowd the horizons of people's lives everywhere, encircling them with the futility of a life unfulfilled, spent in the dusk of decreased human potential.

Your intuitive and psychic abilities can help you open doors, but only to the common ground of the human mind. The semiotics of the commonplace is found in that shared ground. Semiotics, it is often assumed, are the keys to a bigger reality that lurks behind the surface of the ordinary. Nothing in this world is as it appears. A submerged whole is larger than the point that bursts through the deep seas of reality. The symbolic force of our popularly held symbols (for example, "mother") represents the totality of the collective, universal mind, which reveals the truth of our interrelated world.

Being anchored in humility and recognizing that you are part of a much larger total is essential in your meditation practice for accessing the fullest of your capacity to heal yourself and the people around you. Consider yourself to be little. You are a seed going to be planted in rich soil. The chakra of basal survival lies at the root of you, but as you mature, pushing your green shoots through the soil of your conscious mind and into the ethers of higher awareness, you will become not only fresh life, but a strong ecosystem. Your ecosystem, rooted in your enlarged awareness and growing tall and verdant, is a component of the vast ecosystem of universal consciousness. The greater the impact, the taller it grows and the greener its branches become. You will climb to the crown chakra and begin to experience that the leaves on your tree are full of the brilliance of your human potential in every vein and stem. Those leaves and the roots, trunk, and branches they grow are vibrantly alive. Higher consciousness is associated with abundant life. The oxygen that trees supply for us to breathe is similar to what you may provide as a human being who does more than just exist on the conscious level. Eating, drinking, working, and sleeping are the domains of the root chakra.

However, above that level of survival and effort comes something far more rewarding. That item is, without a doubt, sustenance for your spirit. It is nutrition for everything; sustenance nourishes more than you. You are supporting the collective unconscious through your spiritual self-care by creating that spiritual oxygen by keeping the leaves on your branches lush and green. This is why meditation is so crucial. It feeds more people than you. This is the essence of humility practice, which transforms meditation into a portal to a world of love and compassion you've never imagined.

Compassion is the ability to experience the passions of others as though you were experiencing them yourself. Compassion, on the other hand, is much more than an emotion. Empathy is defined as "feeling with." In that emotional environment, compassion is born, and compassion is born to act. Compassion is the identification with what another person is going through and then acting on that shared emotional understanding to effect positive change. Whether the difference is to alleviate poverty, grief, cruelty, or any other form of wrongdoing, compassion is a "praxis."

Compassion is the belief that something should be done to alleviate the situation, as witnessed by the individual who has felt compassion. This is where emotion and cognition collide, resulting in an active solution. That is what the term praxis refers to. It denotes an unavoidable cycle of emotion/thought/action. They complement each other. The birthplace of compassion is the foundation of your contemplative practice in humility. Still, humility teaches you to detach from the ego and judgmental views (culturally required) and cling to a picture of the self as part of something. You are not alone. You are neither an island nor a universe in your own right. You are a part of a whole, and your presence and the quality of that whole matter.

The ego's message is that humans are self-sufficient small islands that exist in a vacuum. The ego is incorrect, and our individuality is at the root of all misery in the world. Everything changes when you recognize how personal your relationship is with the world you view. Most significantly, you have shifted. Only through the ascent of the ego to greater consciousness is such a significant shift conceivable. However, human transformation is at the heart of all change.

We are reaching out to all in utter humility and conscious admittance that we need that connection by detaching from the self and re-attaching to the universal awareness. We already have it, so to put it another way, we reach out in conscious admittance that we need to reconnect. We spark our compassion by reconnecting and being aware of humanity's intrinsic commonality. We can't disregard the whole since we're a part of it. We not only feel it through our empathetic natures (which are also increased by meditation practice), but we also rationally ponder on that emotional reaction before moving beyond feeling to action.

Meditation is an action in and of itself. As I have stated, the tree you are becoming via meditation is life – giving globally. However, your contemplative practice will eventually lead to other actions. You'll feel forced to accept it because you've become a part of something bigger than yourself. It may be an end for individuals who choose meditation as a way of life and spirituality. However, it is simply a small portion of a larger picture for most of us. It is how we discover the fundamental meaning of being human and, as a result, identify our purpose and carry it out in tangible ways. Compassion is our gift to the world, yet simply feeling it is insufficient. Feeling others' pain and difficulties is not the end of compassion. Compassion's ultimate goal is to act to alleviate that suffering and to meet those obstacles. And you're not going to be able to stop yourself. There is no preventing the compassion from flowing out of you once you have reconnected with the entirety of yourself and with the global mind. It will flood your heightened thoughts. It will move your hands, feet, and heart, and you will act out of necessity.

This is not a legal requirement. This naturally occurring generation of praxis arises from the contemplative act. Compassion is a psychic ability. It is the gift of seeing clearly what needs to be done to alleviate the world's suffering and doing it. The meditative practice contributes to this relief. But, like boot camp, meditation practice is not a goal in itself. Your spiritual boot camp transforms you into a compassionate warrior, and warriors charge into combat-ready to gather the injured, heal them, feed them, and love them. Compassion is the true labor that emerges from meditation practice, and it is joy released in action that arises from an open mind and heart. It will become as natural as breathing, just as the messages from your subconscious will become as definite as your conscious mind.

Allowing and Releasing

Releasing is a powerful exercise that may help you awaken your Kundalini energy even more by preventing you from limiting your energy and blocking the area where Kundalini energy wants to flow. We'll look at how you can release even more so that your Kundalini energy may flow even more freely.

Acceptance Equals Flow

Allowing things to happen without instantly falling into a fear-based drive to control everything can be difficult as part of our human upbringing. We tend to want things done a specific way, and we frequently assume that we are doomed if they don't happen the "correct" way. When things do not go as planned, many people may experience a sense akin to a fear of death.

Living in a constant state of dread and the urge to control everything around you is a very terrible way to live. It increases tension and creates a challenging atmosphere for real joy to thrive. It also limits your capacity to enable Kundalini energy (or any energy other than fear) to flow freely.

It is critical to recognize that acceptance equals flow energy when it comes to life and life-force energy. Using flow energy to assist your waking will result in a more profound awakening experience, resulting in less fear. Many people seek to resist as a consequence of fear, and as a result, they directly make their waking difficult. This is because they cannot allow things to flow naturally and instead believe they must control everything.

When you experience pain during your awakening, it is most likely because you oppose energy flow.

Consider shaking a bottle of Coke in your hand. The pressure (energy) within the container would rapidly increase. It would have nowhere to go until you removed the lid. As a result, the bottle would feel bloated and hard to the touch. Consider yourself in this situation. When you choose to awaken Kundalini's energy, you become overwhelmed with energy, and this flow is stopped when you refuse to accept things. Like the coke bottle, you'll have a bloated, rigid sensation that will feel like agony and high energy. You could even feel like a volcano!

It is much simpler to let go of the urge to be in control and let things unfold organically when you accept things. Then, instead of feeling plowed down by high energy accumulation, you may have a more pleasant experience with Kundalini energy.

Steps in Releasing Kundalini Energy

Get Rid of Your Fear

The first step in allowing things to flow is to let go of fear. Fear is the force that pushes us to limit ourselves. When we are terrified of something, we may stiffen up, try to take up less space, and even start trembling. Our bodies become incredibly closed, and our energy becomes even more so. If you are persistently in this state or enter it due to your waking symptoms, you may feel entirely overwhelmed by everything.

Releasing fear may appear complicated, yet it is simpler than you think. Simply lying in your bed once or twice a day and allowing energy to go through you is an excellent method to eliminate fear. Allow the energy to clean out everything that doesn't belong inside you and isn't benefiting you in your experience. This will assist fear energy to leave your body and allow a more positive type of awakened Kundalini energy to flow through you.

When dread arises, simply take a minute to ask your energies to clear themselves. Take some time to reflect on what is going on inside of you. You might even use this as a chance to practice breathing meditation to help you release any energy and relax further. Anything that allows you to let go of fear and choose love and acceptance will benefit your awakening.

Do Away with Daily Expectations

Many of us wake up with preconceived notions about how our day will unfold. When our expectations are not met or things do not go as planned, we become highly unhappy and agitated. This is unneeded stress that can be easily avoided by letting go of everyday expectations.

Take stock of what "needs" to happen when you get up in the morning. For example, you could need to go to work or a doctor's appointment. Then, let go of all other expectations. Let go of expectations about how those activities would unfold. Let go of assumptions about how traffic will be if you remember to bring everything and what will happen. Allow yourself to hope for the best and try your best but let go of the idea that everything will go smoothly every time.

That way, when you undoubtedly suffer daily "annoyances" that everyone does, such as losing your keys in the home and having to rush back for them, getting delayed in traffic, or arriving at the incorrect office for your appointment, you won't sense a substantial increase in tension in your body.

When things unexpectedly happen, as they usually do, you allow yourself to be more open and relaxed, which results in you feeling a lot better. Then, you may relax and enjoy your day because you are not in a near-chronic state of tension. Furthermore, Kundalini energy has a lot more fluid capacity to flow through you since you no longer switch back and forth so quickly between tense and relaxed.

Say Goodbye to People Who Cause You Anguish

One of the most difficult aspects of waking for many individuals is letting go of people in their lives. You've been hanging on to many individuals in your life that don't fit. When we are not working from an awakened state, many of the individuals we tend to maintain in our life are poisonous to us. Even though we love them or feel forced to keep them in our lives, they do not have a claim to our connection. You must keep in mind that you owe no one anything. If the person in issue is someone you cannot avoid, such as a coworker or a boss, and there is nothing you can do about it right now, you should avoid contact as much as possible.

Allowing others to take up space in your life in ways that cause you pain contributes to the continuous state of tension that most people live in. You end up limiting your awakening as a result. You invite unneeded misery into your life, leading to even more suffering.

Allowing relationships to terminate organically when they need to is a better solution. Even if it is difficult and you may go through a mourning process, it may be greatly beneficial for you in the long run. Recognize that guarding yourself, your energy, and your space in this manner is not a selfish act. It is an act of self-love, and it will only offer you serenity and happiness in the end.

Also, recognize that we are in a condition of flow. If you are angry because you do not want to let go of toxic family members, understand that it may not be permanent. It's simply because you are doing your best to take care of yourself in the current moment. If these individuals are no longer harmful in the future or the relationship has an opportunity to repair, you may always welcome them back into your life. Remember to let expectations go. Simply let it flow.

Avoid Places that Hurt You

In addition to individuals who can cause you pain, you may discover that you continue to visit areas that cause you pain. These may not be noticeable aches and pains, but if they cause you discomfort or dissatisfaction, you can be sure that they are causing you some level of suffering or agony.

The most prevalent sites that individuals visit that may cause grief in their lives are:

- Excessively crowded grocery stores or stores that routinely offer low-quality meals
- Your place of employment
- A relative's or a friend's home (often due to feelings of obligation)
- The mall or other locations where you "hang out" that make you uncomfortable
- A doctor's or therapist's office in which you don't feel supported by the doctor or therapist

There are plenty of additional locations that you may be able to conceive of on your own. These locations all have one thing in common: they cause discomfort or annoyance. However, we frequently feel forced to continue visiting these locations for one reason or another. While you may be required to visit similar sites, this does not imply that you must visit the precise spots that give you discomfort or unhappiness simply because you have always done so. You can discover a new grocery store that is fun to shop at and sells higher-quality products. Rather than going to areas that do not bring you peace and satisfaction, you can get a new job or employ a new doctor or therapist. You don't have to hang around in locations that make you uneasy.

Finally, we tend to spend a lot of time in these areas because human conditioning drives us to assume that this is what we should do. Then we become dissatisfied and stressed out since these places do not genuinely provide us with pleasure. However, we seldom go to the base of the problem and devise fresh solutions! Take some time to analyze any location in your life that brings you any amount of misery, and then delete or swap those places for ones that offer you joy and happiness.

Eliminate Old Cycles That Limit Your Awakening

Humans are habitual animals. Everything we do is done in a circle or cycles. Recognizing and eliminating these patterns is a powerful approach to free ourselves from harmful processes that no longer benefit our well-being. We empower ourselves to act differently when we take a minute to address these patterns and choose differently. This implies we may start new cycles that are more in tune with our well-being.

Cycles that become habitual are cycles we commonly encounter but do not notice. For example, someone says something to you that reminds you of something a bully from your childhood said to you. As a result, you feel depressed about yourself and your identity. Then you start to feel disempowered. To relieve your discomfort, you may turn to a soothing behavior, such as eating, smoking, drinking, resting in bed, or anything else. Then, after you've taken care of yourself, you return to your normal routine. When the trigger is pulled again later, the cycle begins again.

These cycles have the potential to consume us. Furthermore, they rarely serve us in any manner. In many situations, the cycles themselves are linked to long-ago events. Sometimes we have already recovered from the trigger, but the cycle has become so habitual that we never take the time to let it go and replace it with a new cycle.

Take the time to understand why these behaviors occur and how you may go about diminishing or eliminating them wherever you find them taking place. Releasing harmful patterns that cause unneeded suffering may influence your recovery and Kundalini Awakening.

CHAPTER 10: THE IMPORTANCE OF VIBRATION AND HOW TO RELEASE IT

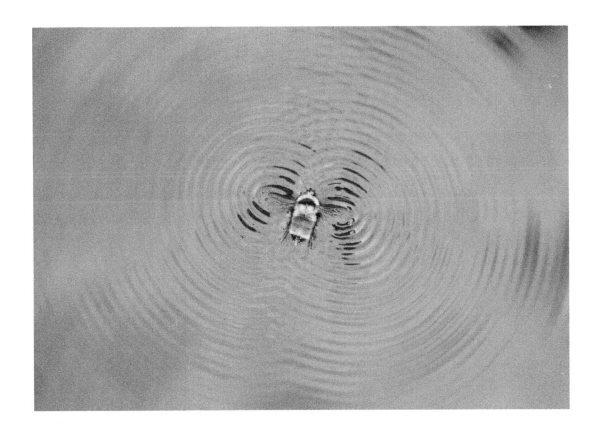

Everything within our planet emits energy, whether or not it is a life force. These energies may frequently radiate up to a foot away from the item they are first bonded to. It is not difficult to see this energy, but it does need practice. We may employ these energies to our advantage in meditation if we recognize that they are all around us.

Many individuals may confuse the vibrating energy of chi with our Kundalini. Chi distinguishes between a corpse and a live human by behaving more like the fire that ignites the flame of life within our bodies. Kundalini is more tied to our souls' energies interacting with our physical bodies. We shall carry our Kundalini's unique energy and awakenings even after death. Chi will no longer exist in our physical existence once we die since death will extinguish the spark of life.

Even though our chi differs from Kundalini in many ways, it is essential to our ascension. There would be no strength for our soul to evolve and awaken on a higher spiritual level if we did not have energy. Understanding the strength of all the forces that fill our cosmos would aid our mental and spiritual development. It is also claimed that anything wrong with or obstructing our chi indicates illness. Clearing one's chi will aid in the healing of diseases and malignancies that impair our physical form, allowing us to feel extravagantly better.

Because chi directly impacts our Kundalini, various strategies have been developed to increase the flow of our chi or life energy, hence boosting the passage of vibrational energies that travel via our Nadi.

There are a variety of exercises we can do to increase the flow of our life force, and tai chi is only one of these effective techniques. Increasing the strength of our chi core so that the fire within us may burn brighter and offer us more energy. Tai chi is a type of dance that assists us in relaxing and visualizing the flow of our energy. One of the major themes of tai chi practice is the ultimate balance of Yin and Yang, making it incredibly popular in the usage of yoga routines across the world.

To practice the traditional instruction of tai chi, one must devote their time to memorizing one hundred and eight hard techniques. These routines have increased our physical balance and flexibility while decreasing blood pressure and cholesterol.

Tai chi has also been linked to an increase in the release of serotonin and endorphins. This practice is well renowned for revitalizing those who employ it. While on the journey of spiritual awareness, strengthening our lifeforce can only lead to success. Knowing how to use the numerous tools and techniques at our disposal is critical to developing our psychic skills.

Depending on the style of meditation we practice or the hardships we are going to encounter, we may build our arsenal of beneficial talismans and energies to aid us in the process. The natural earth components that Mother Nature provides us with are the finest approach to harness this energy. Most rocks and crystals have powerful auras that can help us improve our talents or reduce our threat to others, but any natural creation can benefit us in these ways.

It is generally good to maintain grounding energy on or around us, especially when meditating. These anchoring energies can be found in stones, plants, and animals. These earth entities will also aid in repelling any negativity that may try to enter our auric field.

Sticking to hard stones, crystals, and druses is always a good suggestion for getting the best benefits from this form of energy use. It is also critical that the stone we chose be inside our line of sight in our meditational region, even if it is out of our peripheral vision. These pebbles will make us feel better both physically and emotionally. Stones and crystals operate as containers for energy surges, and these energies may be mirrored back and forth from person to stone.

When a stone reflects too much of us, it can be an unpleasant experience to utilize it for healing. This sort of poison is created by "overload" in our crystals and is readily remedied by a crystal cleansing. A variety of methods may accomplish stone and crystal cleansing. The most well-known is to place the stones under the sun, or better the full or new moon, to recharge and cleanse the energies. Several books and teachings are available that focus on each rock and all of the benefits they may provide to our spiritual progress.

The earth is entirely made up of vibrating energy from its core. One of mother earth's many gifts of enlightenment and healing is the ability to access these energies and forces. We may always turn to the soil and its gift of life to assist us in shaking loose the blocks, preventing our vibratory energy flow. Distinct rocks emit different vibrations, each with its therapeutic properties. It may be difficult to pinpoint the energies we need to work with, but we can never go wrong as long as we allow the stones to call out our auric energies.

A wealth of literature is accessible to assist catalog all of the stones and crystals available to man and their therapeutic abilities. These recommendations can help us narrow down exactly which regions of our energy we wish to repair. It's also a good idea to look for stones that resonate with the hue of the aura we're seeking to remove. Our sixth chakra, the heart chakra, is deep green; green stones can stimulate this energy and encourage good healing.

The more natural and intense the energies, the rawer the stone. Human hands tamper with many stones and jewels, making them smoother and more visually attractive to the naked sight. This does not indicate that the stone's healing properties have been destroyed but that they have been slightly dampened so that their effects are not as potent. There are several methods for "recharging" these stones by utilizing the powers of the earth, sun, and moon. Leaving stones in the rays of a full or new moon helps to charge their vibrational energy significantly.

Smudging and cleansing negativity within or around our stones with dried white sage is also good. Keeping children around plants will also assist in raising their vibrational energy, so having a small indoor garden is excellent. Using dried herbs and flowers can also help with the waking and healing of our spiritual energy. Keeping a pouch of dried lavender at our sides improves our ability to view spirits on the other side. Using lavender oils and flowers throughout our workouts can aid in relieving anxiety and tension and physical skin irritations. Rosemary is also a helpful herb since it serves as an antiseptic. This herb may be utilized to aid in releasing our mental talents and the promotion of spiritual purity.

Vibrational Energy Crystals

The following is a more extensive list of crystals and their benefits:

- **Amethyst** — Gives spiritual protection, cleansing, and well-being
- **Blue Tiger Eye** — Relieves stress and gives emotional balance and clarity
- **Black Obsidian** - Promotes healing, protection, and grounding
- **Azurite** — Enhances communication and intuition while also providing advice
- **Celestite** - Aids in celestial communication, clarity, and the manifestation of our Divine selves
- **Rhodochrosite** - Brings comfort, compassion, and love
- **Bloodstone** — Physically and emotionally detoxifies, promotes healing and grounding

- **Seraphinite (Serafina)** - Assists us in attaining Divine ascension and connecting us to the Devic kingdom
- **Spirit (Cactus) Quartz** - Brings about spiritual connection, oneness, and harmony
- **Selenite** — Enhances our Divine connection and raises our vibrations
- **Hematite** – Extremely grounding and balanced; detoxifies both the body and the psyche
- **Picture Jasper** – Encourages self-assurance and creative vision
- **Sandstone** – Promotes creative, mental, and spiritual clarity and brings us all together
- **Petrified Wood** — Provides stability and strength, as well as grounding energies

Many of these stones may be obtained in most jewelry and rock stores. The higher positive vibrational energies will be present in stones that have not been treated or placed through human-made technologies to "beautify" them and give them a glossier appearance. This is not to suggest that polished stones will not supply vibrational healing energy, for every stone from Mother Earth contains Kundalini power and energy.

Kundalini is a type of vibrating energy. We can use various stones and crystals to assist her in awakening from her rest. The most straightforward technique to determine what type of stone we require is to notice which one we are naturally drawn to while shopping in stores or natural settings. Our body's energies will seek out those it needs, and if we listen, we can uncover some valuable tools for our meditation.

Stones in the form of jewelry are extremely beneficial because they physically surround our aura with various vibrations, which may protect us against negativity and boost our aura.

Creating a balanced meditation environment will be incredibly useful to our Kundalini Awakening process, as long as it is a place that provides us tranquility and peace. Some individuals prefer to be in the company of others by attending Kundalini yoga courses, but others attain a far higher level of awakening when they are alone. While it is not recommended that we force ourselves into difficult circumstances, it is always a good idea to test our limitations and push the boundaries of our comfort zone. We can learn new strategies to help shake the locked gates of our spiritual channel by doing so.

These materials are not required to be included in our meditation, but they might benefit our spiritual recovery.

If we don't have a specific meditation location in mind, we may rapidly create a tranquil setting on our own. Many individuals, for example, prefer to meditate in the warm waters of a bath or shower since it provides a lot of calm and seclusion while also naturally relaxing the body.

It is always a good idea to fill the space with various stones and crystals wherever we choose to construct our meditational setting.

Vital Plants for Meditation Space

Plants are extremely healthy and detoxifying to have in our meditation space. They not only aesthetically relax our minds, but they may also filter the air, which is critical for breathing exercises.

White sage is extremely detoxifying and will protect us as we begin on our road of waking. Smudge and purify the energy inside our auric field using dried white sage. This cleaning power will assist us in getting rid of any bad attachments and energies that may be impeding our healing. As one faces the hardships of waking, healing might make one feel exceedingly vulnerable. Smudging and cleaning our aura will assist us in maintaining a more stable mind and focusing on mending our emotional, physical, and spiritual traumas.

The following are a list of vital plants:

- **Spider Plant** – Purifies the air by removing carbon monoxide
- **Rosemary** – Increases cheerfulness, memory improvement, and tiredness relief
- **Fennel** – Bravery and strength
- **Chamomile** – Aids in healing
- **Marjoram** – Protects and brings enjoyment
- **Lavender** – Reduces anxiety and stress, lowers the heart rate, and cures headaches
- **Ivy** — Cleanses the air and reduces asthma symptoms
- **Basil** – Generates oxygen while absorbing pollutants from the air
- **Oregano** – Promotes happy and healthy family ties and spiritual cleansing
- **Dracaena** — Boosts self-esteem, cleanses the air, and helps us focus our physical and spiritual minds
- **Ficus** – Represents togetherness and understanding; it also represents peace
- **Jasmine** — Opens the heart chakra, increases energy, helps productivity, and elevates self-esteem
- **Lily** – Purifies physical, mental, and spiritual ailments; perfect for a bedroom atmosphere since it promotes relaxation
- **Sage** – Encourages the flow of good energy and eliminates negativity
- **Orchid** – Adds pleasant energy to the home, promotes spiritual well-being, offers oxygen, and promotes romance
- **Money Plant** – Brings prosperity and good fortune, relieves tension, and absorbs synthetic chemicals in the home

These are only a handful of the many plants that might assist us spiritually. If we have pets, be sure that none of the plants we collect are dangerous to them. For instance, lilies are incredibly poisonous to cats, so it's best not to have them around if you have a cat. If we have animals that can access our houseplants, it is much safer to stick with the herbs because they are always safe for our pets to eat.

It's also important to remember the potency of essential oils derived from plants. We can use these oils for their therapeutic medicinal qualities. Many people may turn to the tried-and-true Bach flower remedies because they are high-quality essential oils with powerful vibrational properties. Mixing different plants and oils is also an excellent way to create specific plant-derived tinctures that help our condition. While some may be skeptical of essential oils' therapeutic abilities, the proof will be in the form of improved health.

The lavender plant has been studied as an anti-anxiety and muscle relaxant, but it also has spiritual significance. Having a pouch of dried lavender on hand improves our third-eye vision and allows us to see and hear spirits more clearly.

We may benefit from vibrational healing characteristics as long as we comprehend the earth's powers and the impacts they can have on us. Certain animals can even assist us in our awakening lessons. As long as we are open to receiving their advice, we have numerous guides at our disposal. Suppose an animal keeps appearing in our lives, whether physically or in the form of a photo or a name, then, in that case, we can investigate what messages this particular being is attempting to teach us.

Signs of crickets, frogs, and toads, for example, might signify leaps ahead in our lives and spiritual healing. Frogs and toads also teach us about transformation and change in our lives. A wide range of material is accessible to us focuses on the energies and teachings of the animals and insects that come into contact with humans. Messages from the earth's organisms are valuable gifts and should be regarded as such.

CHAPTER 11: SPIRITUAL ENLIGHTENMENT

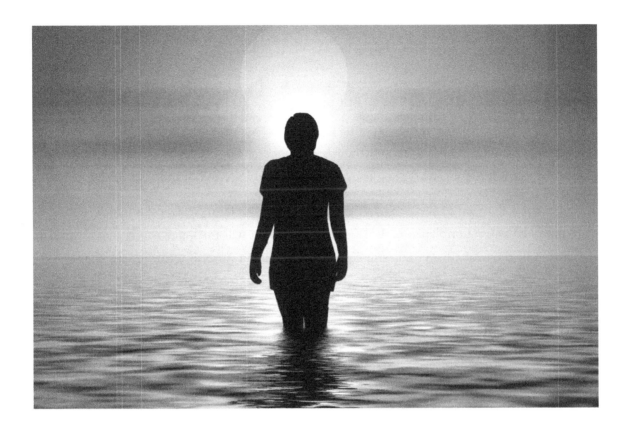

What exactly do we mean when we talk about Enlightenment? Isn't it the flowering of existence for a real seeker of otherworldliness? When one reaches the stage of Enlightenment, one's existence makes a full circle. Looking for Enlightenment in the present era (the metallic age, also known as Kali Yuga in Hinduism) is more unusual than wishing to achieve it in the present lifetime.

What is it difficult to achieve while continuing on the path to Enlightenment? When Swami Vivekananda could have attained Enlightenment under the guidance of his otherworldly ace and heavenly being, Swami Ramakrishna Paramhansa, he didn't! Why?

Illumination (or self-acknowledgment) is the pinnacle of all we recognize as otherworldliness. There is nothing more for an individual to achieve after reaching the stage of Enlightenment. Edmund Hillary was depressed after reaching the summit of Mount Everest because he realized that a great goal had come to an end.

A flower that has sprung loses its importance. It is no longer associated with the plant that gave it life and all that the bud anticipated blooming into an all-out. The value of one's character, sense of self, and self vanished when the bud flowered into magnificent bloom. For as long as the general public smelled the bloom's beautiful perfume, it received recognition. The minute it wilted, no one cared. That's because life moves on and doesn't stop for anyone.

The essence of life is to keep moving forward until one reaches Enlightenment. Furthermore, Enlightenment is the state of being fully free of all that we refer to as the materialistic world. Realism is a physical world marvel. Despite popular belief, Enlightenment remains rooted in the raw reality of human existence. It is simply associated with our own interior identity - our essence (our genuine self). Furthermore, the need for the body vanishes the moment our spirit recognizes and realizes its final potential.

Each illuminated soul must leave the body forever...the cycle of life and birth must end for this enlightened human. If I say that only two people have attained Enlightenment in the last 150 years out of the 6000 million people who live on Earth...then Swami Ramakrishna Paramhansa and Maharishi Ramana were truly honored by God Almighty to have attained Enlightenment, when the general population is directly experiencing such a terrible stage on the worldly plane. Everything is eventually valued in terms of monetary successes.

A highly edified individual living in the deep dark backwoods of the Himalayas today would not find as much unreserved gratitude as any resemblance of Bill Gates – one who will not have the choice of passing on the wealth they manage to the next life yet continually appears to linger around until the last picture of existence arrives. The false belief that money can provide the best in life in the present and after death is a complete myth.

Obstacles of Enlightenment

Some of the primary reasons why people on a spiritual journey may lose out on the potential to live an awakened or enlightened life are as follows:

The Imperative of Understanding

When individuals lack insight about what they are looking for, it is easy to become diverted by some of the spiritual journey's occurrences. This is especially true if you live in a culture that values uniqueness and monetary success. These same aims are applied to the spiritual quest; thus, a person genuinely looks for what is not found in waking.

Another source of confusion is that many spiritual systems have exalted their founders to the point where they are seen as supernatural heroes and saviors of humanity, holy beyond all human impulses. In comparison, the rest of us may feel so inadequate that we do not pursue the experience of realization because we believe we do not deserve it or cannot achieve it. We regard it as some divine grace bestowed onto a virtuous person as compensation, conferring magical abilities, endless life, and psychic insight into the essence of all things. We view the essence of freedom to be intense mystical experiences and unnatural alterations in our capacity or capacities.

It is a great privilege to meet someone awake and living an ordinary life since there is a model we can follow and comprehend outside of our ordinariness. Because awakening is tied to the consciousness that runs through everyone, it may come to everyone. It is a shift in perspective that results in peace, compassion, love, appreciation, and the cessation of confrontation with life. This results in the freedom to express oneself in whatever way one feels driven to express oneself, without being self-conscious, without hesitation, and without becoming trapped in patterns of personal conditioning. The benefit of having an awakened instructor is the modeling that they may give. It is not that you should live your life in the same manner as this individual, but that you may understand that if this person could achieve freedom, so can you.

Too Soon to Stop

When you have a tremendous spiritual or energy encounter and assume it is the conclusion of your trip, you might be rapidly led into a spiritual dead-end.

Adyashanti once stated that following intense awakening experiences. He spent five years with an inner voice telling him, "This is not the end...keep going." This urged him to return to his meditation practice repeatedly.

The accomplishment of the road to enlightenment does not include a continuous overpowering mystical experience, nor does it involve permanently dropping out of the body into some other-worldly existence. It is the abolition of all divisions, the tranquility that comes with understanding that everything is precisely OK. Awakening removes the need to have more, be more, or do better and replaces it with the deepest calm possible. It's as if every movement of the particular "me" has burnt itself out, and one is no longer motivated to relive the past or achieve the future, preferring to live in the now. This settling brings clarity, knowledge, and compassion, and the path of life becomes more natural. Movement is more like a river or a wind, with no connection to the outcome.

If you stop short of this state of being, you may become a spiritualized personality, knowing how to have mystical experiences yet feeling incomplete and uncomfortable. You may fall victim to the "I had it, and now I've lost it" mentality, or you could spend most of your life withdrawing into meditation and avoiding experiencing your experiences. Don't stop until you've gotten rid of yourself. On the other hand, after you've determined that you've discovered the Truth, don't bring every last bit of personal conditioning into the light of day. Allow the process to bring forth what is required and just meet it.

With Ecstasy, Enchantment

Enchantment with some of the byproducts of spiritual seeking – new powers, capabilities, dedication, happiness, altered moods, or self-aggrandizing – can also obstruct the conclusion of a spiritual awakening process. It is lovely to appreciate the gifts that come our way and investigate their depth and expression, but keep in mind that what is most important is understanding who has the experiences. When this is fully understood, all experiences, including those that are not pleasant, strong, or expansive, become acceptable. You become nothing more than the being, the experiencing, and the One who has no propensity to grab or reject any aspect of existence. So, instead of getting hooked to and captivated by one part of life experience, you discover appreciation and pleasure in numerous experiences and acceptance in uncomfortable areas.

Allowing oneself to feel exceptional is how your own experiences may weaken you. A basic ego activity permits hubris to emerge after a deep spiritual breakthrough. If one's intellect is exceptionally creative, it may temporarily lead one down the path of "saving the world" or recruiting followers, in the naïve conviction that you have glimpsed the truth and are ready to lead the masses. It may allow you to discreetly feel superior to others while ignoring the fact that you are no different than them as a human being, utterly conditioned and susceptible to misunderstanding.

Crushing these ideas typically does not work to conquer them. Instead, we must understand our sensitivity to conceit, specialness, and whatever other old self motions surface and choose not to act on them. It is only through loving acceptance of our shadow qualities that we are liberated from subconsciously being influenced by them, and we acquire insight into the limitations of being human.

Doubts

Doubts regarding the potential of being free, or even the reality of freedom, may develop. Our society discourages inner labor and the breakdown of personal egoic inclinations. We witness people obsessed with riches, celebrity, power, sexuality, and even violence. It appears odd to us to live a life that just goes with the flow of things and is unconcerned about a personal acquisition. When we recognize that the price of knowing the Truth is the release of our conceptual frameworks, personal motivations, and old habits, we may believe that this is impractical, not worth the effort, and unlikely to provide any results. And we don't even know if there will be something valuable to take their place when we let go of our attachments. It may lose its attractiveness when freedom is no longer about having things your way but about behaving following some hazy, intuitive, and mysterious truth.

We can capitalize on the emerging uncertainty as long as we don't let it sidetrack us from the process. It can raise important questions and difficulties that lead to a better understanding of who we are. When our behavior falters, or we fall back into an old bad habit, we may begin to doubt our worth. This is an opportunity to uncover buried and unmerged identity patterns that must be brought into consciousness, questioned, and released. Is it true that these beliefs are correct, or are they simply conditioned assumptions?

Discouragement

Discouragement is a common byproduct of spiritual seeking — the sensation that you no longer fit in, can't operate the way you used to or are going through challenging or life-altering physical or emotional situations. Depression, worry, fury, sadness, and all other feelings may emerge for some time after awakening, and a few people may be taken into such despair that they abandon the path. During these night experiences, you may feel a feeling of failure, inadequacy, disappointment, and resistance, and you may lose the spirit to do the inward work requested of you. This is a critical time not to lose hope and explore new depths inside yourself.

It is surprising to find this component of the spiritual path since it defies assumptions. Sometimes, the heart is being forced to shatter, and there is often a sensation of carrying the world's weight. We mourn the end of all conflicts. We share the fury of people who have been displaced. We sense the world's neediness. However, if we can let this pass through us and remove it from our energy field, we will discover quiet beneath and the capacity to continue on our spiritual path.

Many spiritual searchers get enamored with an ashram, monastery, or guru and give up their life in devotion to what they mistakenly believe to be the perfection of that person or institution. In doing so, individuals may overlook clear symptoms of inauthenticity, truth distortions, and even abuse. When a person gets disillusioned and quits a spiritual group, it may feel that their entire universe has fallen and everything they have ever believed has been proven wrong. Recovery might take years.

However, suppose one can accept the collapse as a necessary part of the personal spiritual journey, grieve the losses, establish a personal version of a balanced existence, and gain faith in one's inner wisdom. In that case, this tragedy may become a gateway to freedom. The knowledge and joy formerly known in spiritual practice do not need to be lost; instead, they must be freed from projections on the instructor and group. This is not an easy route, but it has the potential to shatter one's spiritual identity and expose one's heart to freedom. True awakening occurs within us, and no one else can give it to or carry it for us. Worshiping or servicing the impulses and desires of another person does not earn it.

Distractions

Romantic encounters, interesting new jobs, family problems, challenges, illness, the need to earn money, and other events in everyday life draw many people away from their goal of awakening or liberation. This is why, to pursue spiritual activities, it was frequently necessary to give up the world and live in a monastery, retreat center, or ashram. People in certain traditions continue to withdraw for up to three years, unable to leave even when a family crisis arises, to devote their entire focus to spiritual practice. Most genuine spiritual systems are founded on discipline and well-established practices. However, I believe that many of these diversions result from the unraveling of ancient samskaras (inherent conditions) that must still be played out over a lifetime. When we have a genuine hunger for the truth, it will return and guide us toward greater growth when the time comes.

The Fear of an Empty Mind

Our lives are brimming with opportunities for revelation. After all, it is only our truth, the place within us, as eternal, complete, and whole as the ocean. According to non-dual sages, Enlightenment is like being a drop of water and merging into the ocean, knowing "I am this." However, our mental image of Oneness is that it entails the collapse of "me," a loss of boundaries, and a dangerous relapse to childhood or dementia. This is our Western understanding of life without thought, and it is the source of our anxiety about feeling empty.

Every night, we willingly stop thinking about sleep, are unafraid of letting go of ourselves, and are even irritated when sleep does not come. We realize that we need this emptiness to function the next day. Some awakened people experience peace of mind and freedom from thoughts similar to that of sleep, but the clarity of the present heightens it. It is "knowing" without knowing and being able to calmly respond and savor the moment. It is the freedom from constructing words to describe oneself or connect with others, the freedom of being undivided.

Not everyone who wakes up lives in silence the way Eckhart does, and he is certainly an introvert. Even more than Eckhart, the guru Ramana Maharshi lived quietly, and it appears that he rarely had anything to say. However, an awake person may sometimes emit the radiant calm of no thinking. Spiritual searchers frequently respond with this, experiencing it as love or happiness while in its presence, even going into samadhi levels.

If we want to live an awakened life, we must accept emptiness, fall into it with abandon, and grasp its full potential.

The Path to Enlightenment

When one who has been illuminated speaks, there are some things he can say with relative certainty - as much certainty as is imaginable while still in a body in this world. He can say various things with tremendous strength, but not with certainty. There are extra things he could wish to say, but they are significantly more theoretical - not without worth, but susceptible to much larger debate and comprehension of significance.

It is quite beneficial for a master to identify which amount of strength is associated with the articulations that they produce. This is especially important if the master is regularly in and out of the lighted state rather than the enlightened state. Explanations are given when the edified condition may be made with certainty. Explanations based on recalling what was seen and known in the enlightened state communicate an enormous position, but not a certainty. Even a master talks conceptually about strategy and procedures for assisting others in achieving enlightenment, regardless of whether they are illuminated. Nobody, not even the most enlightened teacher, can explain how any other person may take up a section to the hover of enlightened animals.

All lighted individuals speak the same thing; they just communicate in a different language. To go from where you are to where you need to be, you must go through 10 phases. You won't have moved an inch by the time you arrive.

There is just one thing. There is only one problem. There is just one configuration. We now know what we need to do.

1. You become aware of a longing for something more. "Is this all there is?" you wonder. "Most certainly, there must be something more than this," you conclude. You've taken a big risk.
2. You become aware of the concept of lighting. It's only one of many intriguing ideas running through your head.
3. You round the bend and begin to understand that enlightenment is real. This is the third and last step. You're curious; you want to learn more. You start to think about lighting. You start talking about it with others. You start reading books on illumination.

4. You begin to feel the urge for self-edification. The hunger becomes more substantial within, yet it remains mostly in your thoughts. Although this is the fourth stage, it is, in some ways, the true beginning, the beginning of the genuine.

5. You begin your extraterrestrial mission. The dynamic hunt for illumination begins, but you have no idea where to seek it. You have no notion what it is, and you have no idea where to find it. This is the fifth phase; it is both exhilarating and shocking. Your heart joins the chase; you become aware of a deep longing in your heart to return home. You look into various unearthly practices.

6. Your question is directed at the world outside of yourself. This is the sixth and last phase. You may begin to make changes in your life, such as how you live, where you live, who you live with, your career, and so on, but nothing you alter on the planet can satisfy your deep need for something greater. You get perplexed, disillusioned, and overwhelmed; you need to pause and return to your usual life, becoming increasingly familiar and comfortable.

7. Finally, after a long period of research and seeking, you realize that the lower cannot order, the higher; you realize that you have been looking in the wrong place – outside of yourself – and that you can't get illuminated that way. No powerful practice can generate illumination. You cast an inside glance at yourself. You realize that what you are seeking is what you are looking for. Your mind begins to observe itself. You surrender to your higher Self; you let go of the inquiry, yet you have an especially important, deep desire to awaken despite all. You continue your deep quest, but your training has improved significantly. You have selected one meaningful practice from the vast smorgasbord of consequences. Rather than a pursuit, it is more like a supplication of great value, a present to God in acknowledgment of your want to honor him, to remember who you are. This is the seventh and last phase.

8. You just wake up one day. The fantasy of detachment's veil is lifted. You comprehend that you are God; you are the one and only. You see that there is only one thing, and you are it in every way. The eighth phase is your clenched hand arousing. It lasts for a short period, a couple of hours or less, possibly a few days or weeks, but then it fades, and the more common feeling of self-focused awareness returns. You are very troubled by the loss of this ideal light, love, truth, and knowledge. Regardless of your suffering, you have just defeated death; you recognize that what you are cannot die, just your physical body.

9. Your life has now been altered. You live in the present moment, not in the past or the future. You continue on your meaningful path. Your pain is palpable. You stay surrendered in a casing of certainty, with an internal knowing that you will return to that edified state — regardless of whether it is just now of your bodily demise. You continue your inward task of rising above the conscience, healing past wounds, and devouring accumulated karma. The ninth phase is reawakening - the brilliance returns. You are now thoroughly certain; you are not pompous or greedy, and you are no longer scared of anything — there is no fear. You just know who you are, what everything is, what everything isn't, what everything indicates, and what you are to do.

10. The tenth step brings enlightenment to a close. You're always present. Your current duty is to assist others in doing the same.

5 Steps to Enlightenment

Shaktipat

The first step to becoming enlightened is shaktipat. Shaktipat, also known as Kundalini Shakti, Deeksha, or grace, is the profound vitality that stirs you to insight.

Although profound practice and reflection are important if you want to be illuminated, this otherworldly vitality drives you to enlightenment. When this Shaktipat awakens in you, you may experience feelings of ecstasy, love, or harmony. Shakti cleans your vitality channels and stirs you into your natural edified state by allowing your thoughts to remain in that delight.

The most common way to obtain shaktipat is from an edified master, someone who has attained such an elevated level of illumination that they emit shaktipat. Simply sitting with them awakens this otherworldly vitality in you, and illumination occurs.

However, there is another way to obtain shaktipat through sound, which we will discuss near the end of this article.

Purification

The next step in becoming enlightened is refinement. In general, a healthy eating regimen and regular exercise are important. You must get your body into a completely adjusted and unadulterated state. If you drink alcohol, take medications, or eat poor-quality food, your body will be preoccupied with fighting these poisons and remain lopsided. You should eat unadulterated nourishment, heaps of crisp leafy foods, nourishment that nourishes both the body and the mind.

Spiritual Practice

The third method is to engage in the otherworldly practice. Meditation is the most important practice, but Prana (breathing exercises), recitation, and yoga can also help. It is critical to keep an open mind, experiment with the various otherworldly practices discussed by experts, and see what works for you.

Discipline

The fourth way to become illuminated is discipline: to find the profound practices that you find beneficial and to practice them consistently.

You should do what works for you but sticking to a routine gives you energy. For example, I like to get up early, run, do yoga, Pranayama, puja, and recitation, and think before doing anything else. Then I meditate again before supper and again before going to bed. If you want to be enlightened, you must cultivate this vitality and not allow yourself to succumb to apathy and interruptions. I would argue that the option of simply "doing whatever you want" does not work. It only leads to misery and awkwardness. Without a doubt, you should be able to have a fantastic time. Regardless, maintaining this control will help you maintain an illuminated state of mindfulness.

Surrender

The final step to be enlightened is to surrender. Once that profound vitality current is effectively flowing through you due to decontamination, shaktipat, and reflection, all that is left to do is give up and recognize yourself as you are, allowing yourself to feel what is here as a sensation. Although control is necessary when you reach the point where you must stop attempting illumination, the shaktipat drives you to enlightenment. When you experience shakti as a constant in your life, you surrender to it and let it do its work. You permit yourself to experience ecstasy.

CHAPTER 12: MEDITATION EXERCISES

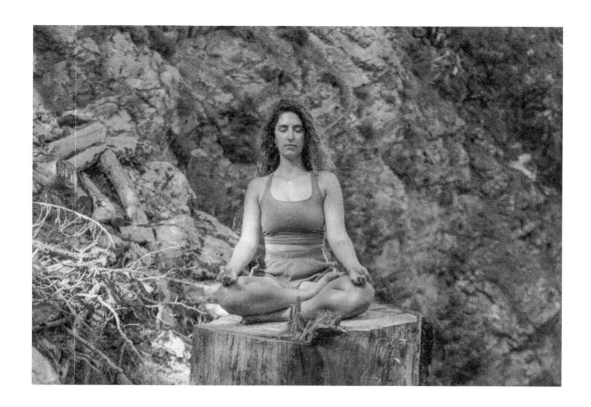

1st Meditation Exercise

Set yourself up in a comfortable position where you will not be disturbed. Close your eyes and take a deep breath for the count of 4, hold for 2 seconds, then exhale for the exact count. While inhaling, tell yourself, "I'm breathing in." Say, "breathing out" as you exhale. Repeat this cycle six times, concentrating on your breathing.

All of your attention should now be on your feet. Our feet work tirelessly for us throughout the day, so we appreciate them for everything they do. Imagine a dazzling, silvery, white light flowing into both of your feet, and then relax your feet. You may begin to experience a tingling feeling, but don't worry if you don't; it will come with repetition.

Bring the bright light up to your knees and relax your lower legs and knees. Bring the bright light gently to your groin area, allowing your thighs to relax. Consider your thigh muscles fully relaxing and softening.

Allow the brilliant light to move towards your hips, relieving any groin and hip tightness. Feel the bright light move up to your heart, past your stomach and navel. Allow your tummy muscles to relax entirely. Because we frequently clench and hold a lot of stress in this area, it is critical to relax and let go.

Feel your chest, shoulders, neck, and lower jaw muscles relax as the brilliant light goes up towards the tip of your head. Any tightness in your cheeks and forehead should be released.

Bring the bright light down your arms, past your elbows, and out through your hands. You may get tingling in your hands.

Maintain this level of absolute relaxation while focusing on your breathing. Feel your entire body relax and release tension.

2nd Meditation Exercise

Set yourself up in a comfortable position where you will not be disturbed. Close your eyes and take a deep breath for the count of 4, hold for 2 seconds, then exhale for the exact count. While inhaling, tell yourself, "I'm breathing in." Say, "breathing out" as you exhale. Repeat this cycle six times, concentrating on your breathing.

Assume you are standing at the bottom of a 20-step staircase. Imagine the number 20 in a vast, legible font in your mind's eye. Step down to the 19th step, feeling yourself going more profound as you do so and visualizing the number 19 in your mind's eye.

Continue down the stairs, feeling yourself growing more comfortable with each step. As you take another step, see the number 18.

Relax the muscles in your thighs, release the tightness in your tummy, and relax your jaw. Let go of all the stress in your body.

...17, 16, feel yourself going deeper... 15, 14, 13, 12, 11, notice how heavy your body feels... 10, 9, 8, 7, 6, 5...you are feeling very relaxed now, as you descend further, you experience a deeper state of relaxation...4...deeper still...3, 2...your body feels heavy, you may feel tingling in certain areas of your body...you descend the final step and see the number 1 in large print in your mind's eye...1. Your body is relaxed, and at peace, your mind is quiet, and you feel calm and rested.

3rd Meditation Exercise

Set yourself up in a comfortable position where you will not be disturbed. Close your eyes and take a deep breath for the count of 4, hold for 2 seconds, then exhale for the same count. While inhaling, tell yourself, "I'm breathing in." Say, "breathing out" as you exhale. Repeat this cycle six times, concentrating on your breathing.

Feel your body enter a deeper level of relaxation. Feel your muscles relax and become soft and loose. Feel your body lightening up and becoming weightless. Allow yourself to relax and trust in the universe's safety entirely. Concentrate your attention on your feet and tell yourself:

"My feet and toes are relaxed"…follow this soothing sensation upwards.

"My groin, hips, lower back, middle back, upper back, spine, and shoulders relaxed."

"My stomach, belly button, midsection, chest, breasts, upper arms, elbows, forearms, hands, and fingers are relaxed."

You're feeling relaxed and at ease. Consider how heavy your muscles think; you may feel like you are sinking into the earth, merging with the cosmos.

"My lower jawbone is relaxed, my ears are relaxed, my cheeks are relaxed, my nose is relaxed, my eyes are relaxed, my forehead is relaxed, and my scalp is calm."

Your body and mind are both at ease. Concentrate on your breathing while following the air as it expands your stomach and rib cage before eventually leaving your body.

4th Meditation Exercise

Set yourself up in a comfortable position where you will not be disturbed. Close your eyes and take a deep breath for the count of 4, hold for 2 seconds, then exhale for the same count. While inhaling, tell yourself, "I'm breathing in." Say, "breathing out" as you exhale. Repeat this cycle six times, concentrating on your breathing.

Begin to breathe in a golden, dazzling light as you continue to focus your attention on your breath. Feel your energy grow as you imagine this light filling every corner of your body. As the golden light escapes your fingertips and surrounds itself over your body, feel your hands begin to tingle.

Immerse yourself in a golden bubble of brilliant light. Imagine floating across the sky in your golden bubble as though on a cloud. Your body feels warm and secure, and you feel safe.

The more time you spend floating, the more completely relaxed you will become. While focusing on your breathing, proceed to repeat, on every inhale..."I am light and in love." Inhale for two seconds, exhale, and repeat, "I am light, I am love."

Inhale for a count of five.

"I am light" (2)

"I am love" (2)

Exhale for a count of three.

"I am light" (2)

"I am love" (2)

Feel yourself in a profound level of relaxation. Your body is suddenly heavy, timeless, and comfortable.

CHAPTER 13: ASTRAL TRAVEL

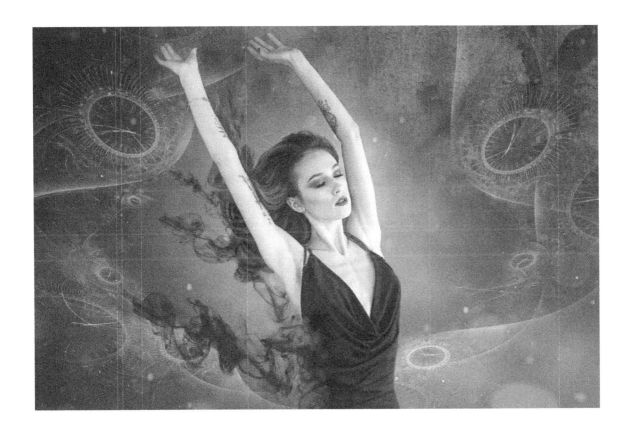

Most people are perplexed by astral travel, yet it is becoming increasingly popular. While many people still find it strange, it's crucial to understand that you and everyone else experience astral travel every time you sleep. Very few people can recall what happens when they travel.

For those unfamiliar, astral travel is the process by which your astral body leaves your physical body and journeys to another location. This is an intriguing skill that will allow you to travel anywhere globally without paying. You can view the Great Wall of China, the Taj Mahal, Ireland, Australia, and other locations. You can even travel to other mystical worlds and celestial realms. This is why so many people desire to learn how to astral travel.

When the issue of astral travel comes up, many people wonder how safe it is. This is a reasonable question. Astral travel separates the physical and astral bodies, but death is just the permanent separation of the two bodies; therefore, it must be harmful, right? No, not exactly. In reality, astral travel is safe. You don't have to be frightened since you've been doing it for years. The only distinction is that you were unaware of it. Learning to astral travel will enable you to do so while also remembering your journeys.

When it comes to learning about astral travel, fear is extremely frequent. I can tell you a thousand times that it is safe, but it's not always easy to believe me. It's hard not to feel scared when you realize you're no longer a part of your physical body. It is only through practice that you will be able to overcome your fear. One of the key reasons astral travel does not function for certain individuals is fear. Fear will lead your astral body to return to your physical body. This is why you must learn how to overcome your fear. You must realize that this is risk-free.

You will be jerked back into your physical body when you feel even the least fear. It is incredibly simple to return to your actual body. All you have to do now is bring yourself back to life. Simply thinking, "I want to be back in my body," will get you there. This is why you must be able to regulate your thoughts. The essential thing is to have a good attitude and avoid being scared. Furthermore, having a bad mentality when astral flying will attract negative spirits. Again, you should not be concerned since you will be returned to your physical body before facing any genuine danger.

Some people encounter the silver rope when astral journeying. This silver cable functions similarly to an umbilical cord in that it connects your astral and physical bodies. This demonstrates that your two bodies are never truly divided. Everyone does not see this silver cord. It's not a huge issue if you don't see one. Don't be concerned if you come across one; just keep on your quest.

You may see your physical body and astral form when you travel, but you may appear as little more than consciousness. You may be able to see or hear what is going on around you. The more you practice this talent, the more proficient you will become.

In the astral realm, you may encounter other creatures or beings. It is advisable not to communicate with anybody or anything in the astral realm while initially starting. They won't disturb you as long as you ignore them. Again, there is no need to be concerned. If you feel threatened, you can return to your physical body. If anything horrible happens, your astral body will be drawn back into your body.

This will allow you to travel to fantastic locations, but it will also assist you in dealing with any worries you may have about dying. Death is just the separation of your physical and astral bodies. It is just temporary with astral travel. This will serve as proof that life continues when your physical body dies.

Most individuals wish to study astral travel because of the numerous benefits. The best part is that anyone can learn how to do it. You must practice, just like you would any other aptitude or skill. Fortunately, you sleep every night, so practicing is simple. The body sleeps during astral travel, but your consciousness remains awake. We'll go through several alternative modes of travel.

Travel Methods

Mental Travel

This isn't strictly astral travel, but it's a wonderful place to start for beginners. Once you've mastered this, you'll be able to go on genuine astral travel. You will just need to utilize your thoughts for this. Your astral and physical bodies will begin at the same time. Depending on how strong your visualization abilities are, this might turn into an astral adventure for you. Take the following actions.

1. Get into a lying-down position that is comfortable for you. Allow yourself to unwind. Take a big breath in and out and relax as if you're about to go asleep. Make certain that your mind is alert and that your spine is straight.
2. Visualize yourself in the room. To see through your closed eyelids, use your mental eyes. Try to glance around your space and pay great attention to the minor features and things you have in it.
3. Consider going out of this room and into the next room in your house. Visualize this chamber in the same way you did the previous. Continue to go through your house's rooms as if you were going to your front entrance.
4. Step outside your door, explore your area and go wherever you wish.
5. When you've concluded your journey, all you have to do is envision the room you're in and think about your actual body. Begin wiggling your toes and fingers, then slowly open your eyes.

This might simply be a visualization exercise, but it is also useful for getting your mind in the right frame of mind. Try to imagine these locations as vividly as possible when doing this. This isn't astral travel because you won't have to envision it while traveling, but it's still a big step in the right direction.

Roll-Out Method

In this method of astral travel, you roll onto your side to separate your two bodies.

1. Prepare to sleep by lying down. Your body will sleep, but your consciousness will remain awake. Allow your body to relax, rest, and sleep by lying down.
2. Feel and think that you are only an astral entity while you do this. Maintain this frame of mind for a few minutes. When you feel linked to your astral body, believing that you are your astral body and not a physical being, you should observe that your physical existence is asleep, but your astral body is awake.
3. You will roll to the side and depart your astral body when you reach this point. If everything goes as planned, you will realize that you are no longer a part of your physical body and are instead of your astral body.
4. Make certain that you do not allow dread to enter your mind. It might be shocking to see your physical body sleeping before you, but you will be dragged back into your body if you get terrified.

5. When you no longer feel linked to your physical body, turn over onto your side. It may be necessary to try this multiple times before you learn the correct sensation or signal for the rolling action. You can roll to either side; the key is that you do it with your astral body.

Floating

In this one, you will float outside of your actual body.

1. As is customary, lie down and rest. Your spine should be straight. Allow yourself to relax by taking slow breaths in and out, but don't fall asleep. Your physical body should be the sole thing to doze off.
2. Feel as if you are in your astral body rather than your physical body. Examine your surroundings with your astral sight. Allow the physical body to relax and fall asleep.
3. When you inhale, you will notice that your astral being will lighten. You will begin to float as you feel lighter. You will initially float above your physical body, then rise higher.
4. Stop focusing on your breath at this time. Concentrate on the sensations you have in your astral body. Continue to float higher by identifying exclusively with your astral body. Move your position to be above your house and floating in the clouds.
5. What types of things do you notice? You have now entered the astral realm. All you have to do now is decide where you want to go. Consider that location, and you will be instantaneously transported there. If you don't have a specific destination in mind, you can simply walk about your area.
6. Consider your bedroom when you wish to go home. When you return to your room, keep an eye on your physical body while it sleeps. Bring it closer to you and input it. Slowly open your eyes and wiggle your toes and fingers.

Third Eye

1. To use this method, you must have an open Third Eye. You will split your two bodies with your Third Eye.
2. Relax by lying down. While your physical body sleeps, your mind stays alert. Your spine should be straight for your energy flow to remain uninterrupted.
3. Try focusing just on your astral body when you're feeling at ease. Take note of how you feel stuck within your physical body. Consider your Third Eye's shimmering azure light to be a portal. This will take you into the astral.
4. Consider your chakra to be a portal to the astral realm. Move your astral body and depart your physical body through your Third Eye chakra.
5. Make certain that you do not feel terrified of seeing your actual body resting there. Because the Third Eye chakra is the chakra nearest to the spirit world, it provides an excellent gateway into the astral realm.

All of these methods apply to astral travel. Choose the one that is the simplest for you to complete. There is no need to master all of the techniques because you only need to employ one at a time. You can also modify these approaches. There are no set regulations that must be followed when engaging in astral travel. Most of the time, astral travel occurs unconsciously, and you only become aware of it after leaving your physical body. These strategies are useful since you may travel on purpose and pick exactly where you want to go.

Helpful Hints

You may do a few things to improve your chances of success when attempting astral travel.

Relax

When you aren't calm, you won't be able to astral travel. The more devoted you are to your physical body, the less relaxed you are. Your body must be so calm that it falls asleep and that your mind remains focused. Don't attempt to conceive of it as astral journeying at first. Concentrate on relaxing your body as if you were about to sleep.

Keep Your Stomach Empty

It is ideal to astral travel on an empty stomach. If you are full, your energy will be split since your body needs the energy to digest your food, so don't do this shortly after eating. Before attempting astral travel, be sure it has been at least two hours since you last ate. A little snack is OK, but not a full meal. You'll need your energy for your journey.

Practice Regularly

It is critical to practice regularly, just as it is with everything else. It's a clever idea to do this every night before going to bed. If you have a habit of falling asleep and losing consciousness, you might want to try this early in the morning. Your body will be rested, making it less likely to fall asleep.

No Expectations

Expectations tend to sabotage astral travel. Let go of your expectations. You shouldn't even hope for success. Expecting anything will sap the energy you need for your journey. It may also result in increased pressure, which will not benefit you. Instead, try to unwind completely. While you may know what to expect when you do this, it is best to forget about it all as you begin your induction. Concentrate on what you need to do and disregard everything else.

Psychic Defense

This isn't required, but it's a nice idea to help assuage any fears you may have and to offer some extra security. The following are some effective techniques to safeguard oneself.

- When traveling, clear your mind of any unpleasant ideas.

- Place a cup of saltwater close to your body or on a nearby table. Negative energy is cleansed and repelled by saltwater.

- Apply some saltwater to your skin before embarking on your journey. This will keep bad energy away from you.

- Make a salt circle around your bed.

- Visualize a white ball of light around your body. This protects you from bad energy.

- Before you travel, say a brief prayer asking for protection.

CHAPTER 14: THE BASIS OF ALL THINGS

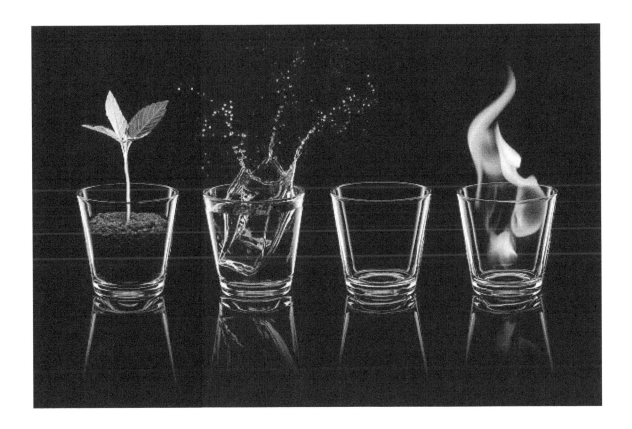

We're going to go over the four elements. These four elements serve as the foundation for everything. We're not simply talking about the physical properties of these objects; we're also talking about their spiritual qualities. These characteristics will allow you to use these aspects to your advantage.

Fire

The element of fire is the first. Everyone has undoubtedly been taught not to play with fire, but odds are the first person to tell them that was a Shaman, not a concerned parent. The Shaman was aware of the fire's ferocity and beauty. It is associated with, among other things, resolve, war, bravery, courage, pleasure, sex, passion, and willpower. The fire has a tangible presence, which might help you recall its attributes.

If you begin to feel terrified or lose hope, you might find power in fire. Fire also relates to clairvoyance, firedrakes, Hestia, midday, manly, cactus, rosemary, south, and salamanders. Working with fire may aid in developing your Third Eye since it brings in light, allowing nothing to be hidden.

Fire has the incredible ability to form your drive and will. The inner light leads you, and the Divine Fire burns within every soul. Like all other elements, fire has an earth plane form and a form in all other spiritual realms. It is an energy source that must be used with caution and care, or you will be burnt, or more accurately, burned out.

You must ensure that you set boundaries for your fire to tend to and feed it. Fire's nature is uncontrolled and combustive, especially when combined with air energy. As a result, when you first begin working with elements, you should begin with earth because it is your anchoring cornerstone.

While fire consumes, it also returns warmth and light. In the dark, it flashes brightly and sparkles.

Fire is one of the four elements associated with force and passion in Greek philosophy. In Greek mythology, a fire was so strong that it required Prometheus to take it from the sun so that humanity may survive, for which the Gods punished him.

Heraclitus, a Greek philosopher, provided insight into fire and its relation to the human spirit. He thought that the soul was made up of fire and water. The everlasting soul wishes to become just fire, commonly seen as enlightenment. This was far from his only observation. He also believed that the universe is always changing, as well as the doctrine known as the unity of opposites, the same as the Wiccan proverb "As above, so below."

Plato was the one who bestowed the sacred mathematical shape of the tetrahedron on fire. He reasoned that fire does not require several sides to reveal its action. Consider the heat of a little cluster of hot embers.

Fire is seen as primal and powerful in far Eastern beliefs. Our metabolism is the physical embodiment of fire. It manifests as desire, personal drive, and intention in mind.

In Hinduism, Agni is a deity who represents the sun, lightning, and fire. Agni serves as a messenger between the earth and the sky, maintains youth, and receives gifts. Fire is a symbol of immortality and communication in this mythology.

Water

Water is the second element. It has a strong connection to emotions, cleaning, beauty, relaxation, and healing, among other things. It is related to the West direction. Try working with the water element when it comes to self-improvement or healing.

Silver, mirror, cauldron and cup, nymphs, undines, sense of taste, inverted triangle, blue, and Aphrodite are all associated with the water element. Crabs, swans, water snakes, dragons, and fish are the animals most intricately connected with water. Any cleaning job that is done must use the element of water.

Water is one of the easiest elements to manipulate. Washing your hands might help to clear your energy when you are worried. When you reheat your water, you are introducing the element of fire. Our tears are saltwater that carries spiritual meaning when we cry. Tears may be used to mark ritual goods and be utilized in potions or anointing things. The essential thing to remember is that whatever feeling you had when you cried will become a part of what you're working on.

Because humans are formed of water, our entire existence resonates with the element of water. All you have to do is become more aware of this relationship. Water can absorb love, and everything done from a position of love is extremely powerful.

Water scrying is a divination method that allows people to use water. This is when you use the water's surface like a mirror. This is best done on a night when the moon is low since the moon regulates the ebb and flow of the water. When you let your eyes wander, the shimmer of the water will transform into a picture. This works best if you already have a question in mind so that the symbols make sense to you. A water bowl will suffice if you don't have access to a lake or ocean.

Air

The element of air comes next. The element of air is related to the direction of the East. Sword, wand, spring, wisdom and knowledge, hearing, scent, dawn, gossip, intelligence, and communication are some of its other connections. Eagles, spiders, and ravens are creatures linked with air. Its hue is yellow, which represents manly vitality. Working with air will assist you in freeing your spirit and strengthening your mind.

Air represents the crucial breath that we all require to survive. Air comes to us in many forms, from the winds that formed the universe to the first screams. Earth is stationary, while air moves.

In Greek philosophy, the air was divided into two parts: the atmosphere in which we dwell and the upper area above the clouds. In Greek philosophy, Aer was the lower atmosphere, whereas Aether was the upper realm. Aristotle even regarded Aether as having created the celestial sphere.

In sacred geometry, the octahedron represents air, alchemically placed between fire and water. The Greeks' terminology for the elements is difficult, but they loved to make everything sound lofty. In layman's terms, this indicates that air energy likes interacting with water and fire, and it may be utilized to build a bridge between the two.

The Hindu term for wind is *vata*, which means to blow. Prana also refers to the life-giving breath. Prana is regarded as a Father God, and his breath is regarded as one of the five holy elements in Hinduism. Air does not exist in Chinese systems. Qi, a spiritual flow and breath, is mentioned in Chinese traditions. Air exists to remind us that there is much more to the world than we can see, and it reminds us that we must evolve and develop in tandem with the rest of the universe.

Earth

Finally, there is the element of earth. This is the one with the closest ties to humanity. You will always be connected to earth because you are constantly in the energy of earth, no matter where you are or what you do.

The earth is associated with foundations, stability, fortune, materialization, prosperity, centeredness, and anchoring. It is a feminine energy that is linked to the direction North. Dionysus, Pan, Arawn, Mah, Rhea, Gaea, Adonis, Athos, and Ceres are all associated. Trolls and gnomes are the creatures linked with earth. Brown and green are the hues associated with the earth. Because we all live on Earth, you must connect with the element.

The bulk of legends involving the element of earth involves spirits that reside in plants or a dimensional place next to your own. Plants, flowers, and trees are frequently cared for by these animals. Some dwell underground and enjoy the Earth without human intervention, while others will mingle with wanderers. Elves are frequently depicted as magical in stories involving them. Some individuals aid good people, while others have their agenda. So, when dealing with Earth creatures, keep in mind that they might be capricious and aren't quite as trustworthy as Mother Earth.

Various parts of the earth might be beneficial when it comes to spirituality. Elemental vibrations include, for example, ley lines, which are power lines. They may be found worldwide, and when they intersect, you will always discover a hallowed site. Some of these crosses include the Callanish in Scotland, where stories tell of ancient dragons staying there to defend the world's stone circles.

Unlike the enigmatic air, earth is a substantial element. When you meditate on earth, you may concentrate on the beauty of healing stones and crystals, the soil used to grow your food, the animals and plants it supports, and see it from space as a reminder of your heavenly Island. Earth energies may help with all types of manifestation by forming strong roots where your aspirations can become a reality.

This is not to imply that the earth is entirely positive. It has the potential to be ferocious. Consider the devastation caused by an earthquake or the devastation caused by an erupting volcano. Because of this power, you must respect Mother Nature.

Making Use of the Elements

Understanding the properties and characteristics of the components is only one part of the equation. The other need is the ability to use the components. There are no fixed rules on any elements' ideal or right traits or features, as they might vary from person to person. A person who is more linked with fire, for example, will find it more calming than water. That is why you must work with the components and get to know them to determine which one works best for you. Still, it's vital to recall their typical characteristics, symbols, and meanings, since these will be items you may rely on.

How Should These Components be Used?

Once you've worked out how each of these aspects impacts you, you can start leveraging them to your advantage in various circumstances. For example, if water helps you feel peaceful, you may utilize water to help you feel less worried or nervous when these sensations arise. Soaking in a tub of water is a fantastic option to accomplish this if you don't have easy access to a natural water source. You may also add salt to your bath water to aid in cleaning.

If you want to improve your willpower, you should work with fire. Simply lying out in the sun will be enough. While you're doing it, imagine the sun's beams energizing you. Make sure you apply sunscreen beforehand. It does not affect the sun's strength and will protect your skin.

If you're feeling uneasy or ungrounded, you need to reconnect with the earth. Many individuals may walk outside barefoot to feel the earth beneath their feet. Feel the earth's strength anchoring you and providing stability.

If you're having trouble moving on from anything, you need to connect with air more. Spending time outside will aid in your connection with air. Feel the wind sweep away your worries and troubles.

When it comes down to it, connecting with the elements and applying them to your daily life isn't that difficult. The most important thing is to get to know them more intimately and understand how they impact you. This will guarantee that you use them as effectively as possible. This has a wide range of applications and variants. You don't have to strive to learn them all since you'll spend more time studying than doing. It is also beneficial to try to create your findings. Proficiency in the elements will do wonders for your life and undoubtedly improve it.

CHAPTER 15: THE AURA

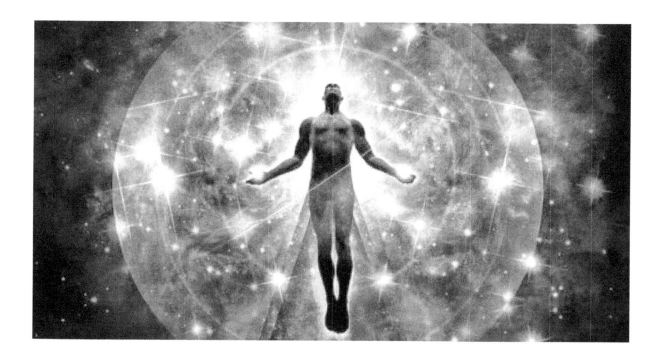

You've heard the term *aura*, but do you know what it entails? A brightness or emission is what an aura is. It's a component of your energy body. Every object in the universe has an aura. Auras may be found in inanimate things, plants, trees, animals, and humans.

Auras may disclose a person's emotions, health, and mental condition. Kirlian photography has been created to depict a person's aura. Doctors have used it to diagnose patients. A person's aura will indicate any ailments or illnesses before they emerge in the body. Kirlian photography will photograph your aura.

There are different methods for determining what is in a person's aura. The ability to read auras is quite useful. You must be able to see or feel them do so. An aura is composed of several levels. The etheric aura is the one nearest to a person's physical body. Other auras include spiritual, emotional, and mental auras, among others.

Observing the Aura

You must first be able to feel an aura before you can see it. There is a way for sensitizing the hands. Grandmaster Choa Kok Sui, the creator of Pranic Healing, taught it. Follow these steps:

1. Make a fist with your hands and rub them together.

2. Place your hands in front of you as if holding a little ball between them. Your hands must be facing each other.

3. Inhale deeply and slowly spread your hands apart. Breathe out and bring your hands closer together, but don't let them contact you. Continue to exhale gently and inhale slowly.

4. You should start to sense a tingling sensation or pressure between your hands. This indicates that your hands have been tuned, and you should now be able to detect an aura.

5. Holding your palm out, you might try to sense your aura. You might also try to sense other auras by heading toward another person or live thing while keeping your palms outward. You should quickly sense a pulling or repelling force. This is the aura of an object or person.

The more you sensitize your hands, the simpler it will be to detect auras. Try sensing the auras of various items and people; you'll be surprised at how different they all feel.

Let us now look at how to see an aura. Auras are easy to detect. You'll need a neutral background and modest lighting. The steps are as follows:

1. Hold your hands out in front of you, palms facing out. Extend your fingers widely.

2. Place your hands against a blank wall.

3. Apply soft focus now. This is gazing at something without really focusing on it.

4. You'll use your peripheral vision to get a better perspective.

Relax and keep staring. Soon, you'll see the light growing around your hands. It may start as white light, but with practice, you will notice various hues such as blue, yellow, and others.

Here's another technique to observe a person's aura:

1. Concentrate on a person's Third Eye chakra while staring at them.

2. Allow your peripheral vision to see the whole body of the individual.

3. You will easily notice the person's aura if you use soft focus. It may start white, but as you practice, you will be able to see additional hues.

The key concept is to learn to use your peripheral vision instead of staring forward. There is no magic at all involved. It is normal to be able to see a person's aura. Contemporary society has taught us that this capacity is unusual, whereas it is quite common and remarkably simple for people.

Colors of the Aura

Let's look at how to interpret aura colors now. A long time ago, clairvoyants were asked to stare at the same individual and interpret their observed auras. They were first disappointed. Colors were seen differently by each clairvoyant. Some people viewed the person's aura as orange, while others saw it as yellow, and so on. They all were liars or imposters. They quickly understood that auric sight is a subjective experience.

Colors perceived varied depending on what a certain hue represents to you. This is why clairvoyants perceive the color of an aura differently. When comparing a person's emotions, state of mind, and health, they all had the same reading. When reading auras, you must consider what a particular hue signifies.

The Mind's Ability

Despite technological advances, the human mind remains a mystery. There is simply too much about it that is yet unknown, especially when considering all of its potential. "All is thought; the universe is mental," says the Kybalion. You will be able to master anything if you can master your thoughts. The bad news is that mastering your thoughts is not simple. This is evident when you attempt to meditate for the first time. When you're first starting, it's difficult to keep your mind undisturbed and motionless for a few minutes. You can tame and manage your thoughts with practice.

You must learn to regulate your mind as part of your spiritual growth since it holds the key to your hidden potentials and abilities. The whole power of the mind has yet to be discovered and harnessed. This is because the mind's capacities are unbounded except what you place on it. Our minds have tremendous power. You must master it.

Increasing Your Influence

How can you increase the strength of your mind? Unfortunately, there are no shortcuts available. The only way to achieve this is to practice constantly. Nothing makes sense without our thoughts, energies, and chakras. You're already familiar with several techniques for increasing the strength of your mind. All you have to do now is keep practicing.

It's critical to understand that the mind's power isn't limited to vision. It is possible to rely on faith. You should believe in all you do. Don't only think of them as methods. You must be able to sense and visualize your energy and chakras. You must understand that you have the power to regulate energy. These aren't simply fictitious tactics for revealing your mind's genuine power, especially if you can harness it while using these procedures.

Don't expect to be able to learn these strategies quickly. Our minds require time to acclimate to new experiences. Don't be shocked if you can't do a certain method even if you understand the directions. As previously said, you must practice, practice, and practice some more. Knowledge is different from being able to perform effectively.

I can't emphasize this enough: if you genuinely want to transform the strength of your mind, practicing meditation will always be a good idea. There is nothing better for mind training than daily meditation practice. The good news is that any meditation is beneficial to your mind, so you may choose which techniques to apply. When you've decided on a technique that works best for you, all you have to do is participate in it and practice it frequently.

Mind-Body Healing

Healing with your mind, often known as mind-healing, is an intriguing topic. After you've learned how to cure yourself, you'll be able to teach others how to heal themselves.

The power of your mind is only as strong as you choose to make it. To be honest, it has no limitations or restrictions. Only you can limit what it can accomplish. Pranic, Reiki, and other healing modalities rely on the power of the mind.

Your mind may be both an adversary and an ally. If you cannot control it, it may cause havoc within you. You must learn to calm your mind and maintain complete control over your thoughts. To paraphrase an ancient adage, "The quality of your life is determined by the quality of your ideas."

CHAPTER 16: ORIGIN OF THE CHAKRA SYSTEM

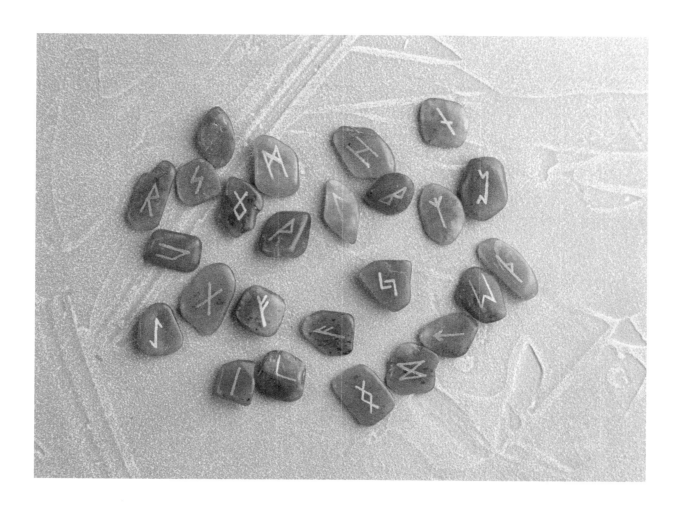

Chakras are energy centers located at various points throughout the body. The term "chakra" is derived from the Sanskrit word "tss chakra," which means "wheel, disc, or cycle." The Rigveda describes chakra as a wheel with several spokes. It is hardly strange, however, that most depictions of chakra depict it as a living, cyclic ball of energy.

Energy is all around us. In reality, everything we see, feel, smell, or hear is made up of energy. This energy manifests itself in many perceptible activities like movement, thought, laughing, emotions, rage, etc. Ancient Indian literature informs us that the gross body (physical body) comprises five components.

These elements, which are also essential components of nature and life as we know it, are known as the mahabhutas, and they include:

- Prithivi or earth

- Jala or water
- Tejas or fire
- Vayu or air
- Akasha or space

The chakra system is based on ancient Tantric literature. Tantra is a significant yet complex nonreligious philosophy. Tantra is an etymological term that means "to weave." As a result, tantra may be defined as a process in which we weave together the knowledge of the body and the strength of the intellect to gain enlightenment, self-mastery, and ultimate consciousness.

Meaning of Chakras

Each chakra may be seen as a spinning wheel within the body that holds the energy of that specific system. There are seven unique chakras, each controlling and maintaining a certain body region and different traits inside ourselves. The chakras are physically placed within the body and serve as a mental and spiritual focal point for us to use in meditation and other energy healing activities.

Many of us recognize that the mind and body interact with one another, impacting how each works. However, few of us comprehend the distinction between the physical body and the mental energy that powers it and how the two systems are intertwined. It is acknowledged in all religions that contain chakra knowledge that there is an energy that surrounds and goes through the body. This energy is known as the "subtle body," which distinguishes the physical experience from the spiritual one. The subtle body refers to a level of existence apart from the physical reality. This plane is spiritual rather than physical, and it is linked to a greater notion, a higher sphere of existence.

Because the notions of the subtle body and many planes of existence may be highly confusing and difficult to grasp, we will concentrate solely on the chakras and how they affect our physical experiences.

While we cannot see the chakras, their effect on our lives may be felt daily. There are seven chakras in all, which create a line from the bottom of our spine to the top of our head. Some religious belief systems dispute the number of chakras, with some claiming only five and others claiming thousands, but the most prevalent interpretation accepts the usual seven.

Working your way up from the base of the spine, you have:

- The Root Chakra
- Sacral Chakra
- Navel Chakra
- The Heart Chakra
- Throat Chakra
- The Third Eye Chakra

- The Crown Chakra

As you can see, each chakra connects to a certain area of the body and significantly influences each of those systems. When the chakras become blocked or imbalanced, it can lead to physical diseases and other issues that negatively influence our lives. It is recommended that each individual understand how to open each chakra and maintain them balanced and flowing to have a healthy and functional mental and physical experience.

You may be wondering what we mean when we talk about opening or balancing your chakras. If you are having difficulties in your relationships, having difficulty sleeping, feeling stressed, or getting ill often, you may have an imbalance in your chakras that contributes to these problems. If you can focus on each chakra, you will be able to understand where you are stuck and the underlying reason for the imbalance. You may correct the problem with numerous workouts and ways to restore healthy energy flow.

Origin of the Chakra System

The chakra system may be traced back many millennia, with the name *chakras* first appearing in the Hindu Vedas. The Vedas, written in ancient India, is among the earliest religious scriptures, dating back to the first and second centuries BCE. Following the Hindu Vedas, chakras were addressed again in the 8th century CE inside Buddhist scriptures describing the body's many energy centers. Only four chakras are referenced in Buddhist scriptures, but this was enlarged through time to include the seven that we know today.

There are numerous connections and similarities amongst the chakras, regardless of whatever tradition you turn to. The notion of a subtle body, sometimes known as a soul in the West, is commonly stated. The subtle body is said to exist while we dream and is what departs our bodies when we die. The chakras are linked to this aspect of our being and govern the health and well-being of our energy rather than our physical presence. While our spiritual body is distinct from our physical body, the two are inextricably linked, and one cannot survive without the other.

This is why both systems have such a large influence on our well-being because any issues in one cause difficulties in the other.

Tantra practice has grown in popularity as the notion of energy centers has grown and evolved. Tantra simply means "connecting and growing," and Tantric yoga is the most well-known kind of tantra practice. Tantric yoga is a method of connecting with and connecting to your spiritual energy, and it is one of many techniques for people to recognize and balance their chakras. Tantric yoga was initially used in the Vedas writings that we reviewed, but it did not become as entwined with the chakras until around 900 CE.

After 900 CE, the seven chakra systems as we know them now began to gain root during the 17th century. At this moment, it began to spread to the West, and in the 18th and 19th centuries, it was taught outside of the Eastern culture in the form of books and new-age instructors.

The seven chakras became the main belief system when the chakra system gained acceptance in the West. These seven chakras weave their way into several different spiritual notions and traditions. Their impact may be seen in Hatha Yoga, Reiki healing, meditation, tarot card reading, and other beliefs and activities. Kundalini yoga, a modern fusion of several yogi traditions, is centered on the notion of the chakras and entails mixing yoga with meditation and chants to balance and open up each person's spiritual energy or chakras.

Regardless of the individual faith, chakra energy has historically been a well-valued topic of study in the current era of spiritual health. Prana in Hindu traditions, Qi in Chinese, and simply our soul by others have all been used to describe the life energy that flows through our bodies. Whatever you name it, most people believe that something beyond our physical bodies makes us who we are, and therefore, the chakras are significant to all of us in that way.

Chakra Energy

So, you're wondering, "How does all of this work?" That's a good question. This material goes beyond what we learn in school or from our parents. It is not taught in traditional classrooms or encyclopedias, and the bulk of us must seek it out for ourselves. You've chosen this book because you're curious yet understanding these complicated topics may be tough and perplexing.

Spiritual energy means different things to different individuals, making it difficult to provide a comprehensive and encompassing explanation of what it is and how it operates. Some believe it is a god or divinity, while others believe it is something that emanates from the ground itself. It is personal to you how you feel it came to be, but what it is may be stated more readily. In some ways, spiritual energy is similar to what you experience when you close your eyes and concentrate on your breathing. You get the actual sensation of your body being alive when chilly air fills your lungs, and then warm air is released. It's also how you could feel when you're alone, have a heart-to-heart with a buddy, gaze at the stars at night, or feel wonderfully overwhelmed by the human experience. Those experiences connect you to your spiritual energy and serve as an excellent beginning point for learning about the chakras.

Working with that energy is what you must learn if you wish to open and balance your chakras and your total spiritual energy. However, before you can work with it, you must first be able to identify and isolate it. To do so, you must first understand how to detect your energy and what to look for in terms of the many feelings that you may experience. Taking the time to be alone with your energy, absolutely free of distractions, is one of the finest methods to learn about it. However, all you need to do for the fundamentals of meditation is sit motionlessly and close your eyes, turn off your thoughts, and focus solely on yourself. Consider the following:

1. Locate a peaceful location where you will not be disturbed.
2. Take a seat on the floor or in a comfortable chair for you.
3. Shut your eyes.
4. Inhale deeply and hold for 3 seconds.
5. Exhale slowly and pause for 3 seconds.

6. Repeat the inhale, pause, exhale, pause procedure.
7. While you're inhaling, think of nothing else, but you're breathing.
8. Allow your thoughts to drift away if they arise.
9. Spend 15 minutes at this moment.
10. Do this every day.

The more at ease you get with being in this zone, the more you will be able to connect with your spiritual energy. Once you've understood and felt it, you may start working with it more intimately. When meditating and tapping into your energy, you may experience the following sensations:

- You may feel physical pain, such as muscular stiffness.
- It may cause mental distress, such as melancholy or guilt.
- There might be a sense of immense emotional release and relief.
- Your body may feel as if electricity is coursing through it.
- You may get a suffocating sensation in your chest.
- Some people notice a temperature shift and get too chilly or too hot.
- Many people discover that a sense of tranquility will overpower them.
- When people's eyes are closed, they may perceive distinct hues.
- Others will have no feelings at all.

Whatever you are going through, realize that it is perfectly normal. Each individual will connect uniquely, and no two people will have the same spiritual awakening. Instead, it is about being more in tune with yourself rather than attempting to mimic what a friend, instructor, or random person has gone through.

What Role do Chakras Play in the Physical Body?

While the chakras are a component of our spiritual body, they also relate to our physical body. The chakras, like other systems, mirror things like our digestive system since everything affects everything else. For example, if you ate something that disturbed your stomach, the discomfort would go down to your intestines, causing a chain reaction that might end in some unpleasant outcomes. The chakra system works similarly in that if one of the chakras is out of balance, it sets off a chain reaction that leads to even more terrible conditions. But, in addition to communicating with itself, how does it connect with the rest of our body?

Our endocrine system is the first main system to which the chakras link. The endocrine system is comprised of glands located throughout the body that operate to control our hormones, which impact digestion, metabolism, growth, sexual function, mood, and other functions. These glands flow straight from our genital area to our skulls, which may seem familiar. Because several of the chakras are placed in the same location as each of these glands, they directly affect their operation. Among these relationships are:

- **The Adrenal Cortex Gland** - How our bodies respond to stress

- **Sexual Organs** - Our sex drive and reproductive functions are represented by the Sacral Chakra
- **The Navel Chakra Pancreas** - controls our blood sugar levels
- **The Thymus Gland** - Produces T Cells for your immune system's response
- **Thyroid Gland** (Throat Chakra) - Affects our metabolism
- **Pituitary Gland** - Secretes hormones and delivers messages to the other glands
- **The Crown Chakra Pineal Gland** - Melatonin production for our sleep cycle

As you can see, there is a direct relationship between the physical body and the spiritual wheel placed at each one, and each gland has a significant impact on our lives. To guarantee that everything in the Endocrine System functions properly, we must also ensure that its mirroring chakra is balanced.

However, it is not only the Endocrine System related to the chakras; the nervous system also has a direct link. The nervous system refers to all of the nerves and cells in our bodies responsible for sending and receiving information to and from the brain. The nervous system is in charge of interacting with our surroundings, gathering all of the sensory information that we encounter in our daily lives. It then gathers all of that information, interprets it, and sends a message to our body, causing it to respond appropriately. For example, if you are cooking and touching a hot skillet, your nervous system will recognize that you have touched something dangerous and that it is causing you injury. It collects the data, sends it to our brain, and waits for a reaction. Our brain tells us that it is hot, that it hurts, and that we should remove our hands. Therefore, the nervous system tells our hand to pull away and tells the nerve ending there that pain exists.

Some of the nerves that make up the nervous system all gather together in a clump at particular points in our bodies, known as plexuses. As you can see from the list, each plexus connects directly to its Chakra:

- **The Heart Chakra Cardiac Plexus** - Sends and receives signals from the heart

- **The Navel Chakra Celiac Plexus** - Sends and receives signals from the stomach, pancreas, and liver

- **The Sacral Chakra Superior Hypogastric Plexus** - Sends and receives signals from the reproductive organs

- **Inferior Hypogastric Plexus** - Supply signals to and from the gut and bladder area

As with the endocrine system, the nervous system may be directly influenced by chakras located nearby and how our bodies work. If we disregard the chakras and fail to balance them, we may face issues beyond our spiritual side.

Awakening the Chakras

You will be able to awaken each of the seven chakras once you have identified and isolated your spiritual energy. Simply meditating starts your road to awakening because you acknowledge and identify the energy that already resides within you. Whether you were aware of them, the chakras have always existed, and ignoring them does not make them disappear. Instead of allowing them to become blocked or imbalanced, the idea is to make them as open and balanced as possible.

We always start the awakening process at the base of the spine, where the Root Chakra is located. Our spiritual energy is housed here, but it is also obstructed and held back from going throughout the rest of our body. When your chakras are blocked or out of balance, you may suffer a variety of symptoms and indicators, some of which are as follows:

- Nightmares regularly and difficulties sleeping
- Panic attacks and anxiety disorders
- Physical discomfort and stiffness in the body
- Feeling a lack of inspiration and creativity
- Depression, as well as a loss of interest and drive
- A decrease in sexual desire and sexual pleasure interest
- Self-esteem and self-worth issues
- Anger problems and a quick temper
- Digestive problems and stomach discomfort
- Frequently harboring grudges and difficult to forgive
- Difficulties establishing and maintaining romantic relationships
- Friendships that are toxic and interpersonal connections that are unsatisfying
- Inability to pay attention to things over extended periods
- Constant headaches and neck and shoulder tension
- Having a negative attitude toward others
- Isolation and a lack of connection with people

As you can see from the list above, the symptoms range from physical to mental and can impact any number of regions of the body and mind. Keeping your chakras balanced can positively influence your life since they affect you in all aspects.

Yoga & Chakras

Vitality and Spiritual Awakening

Each chakra contains numerous levels of energy that work together to contribute to the overall health of the chakras. The chakras are interrelated and operate together as a whole. If one chakra is out of balance, the others around it compensate for that imbalance. To avoid imbalances and blockages in numerous areas, it is essential to pay attention to the chakras and recognize their presence in your body.

In further detail, these imbalances or blocks can appear as a range of unpleasant bodily and mental diseases. Chakra balancing improves the entire energy flow throughout the body, making us feel lighter, happier, and healthier.

The Divine Energy Flow

All day, every day, energy flows steadily through the chakras. It fuels your body and your life. It is in charge of pulling you out of bed in the morning and keeping you active throughout the day. It is our life energy, and it sustains us. We need it to live.

You have free-flowing, balanced energy flowing through your chakras if you wake up energized and ready to face the day. This balance will get you through the day and help you accomplish your objectives, enjoy your life, have satisfying relationships with others, and accept and love yourself completely.

Far too frequently, we find ourselves in physical or emotional distress. While suffering is an inevitable part of life, it does not have to control our lives. We will notice a considerable improvement in our general health and well-being if our energy is freely flowing.

This life force or energy is known as Prana, and when it runs freely through the chakra system, we feel healthy, light, and balanced. Sadly, it's a fantastic sensation that many do not enjoy daily. This is why it is critical to become aware of the chakras within our bodies.

Healing Potential of Yoga

Well-balanced yoga practice may be beneficial for reaching health and wellness in the body, mind, and soul. "Yoga" means "yoke," but it may also mean "unify" or "unite." This unity represents the connection of mind, body, and spirit, which may be realized over time via persistent yoga practice. Well-balanced yoga includes breathing methods, meditation, and asana practice — the physical postures of yoga, which most people think of.

Yoga allows us to renew and rejuvenate our bodies and minds, which aids in connecting with the spirit. Although many individuals practice yoga for weight reduction, injury healing, or relaxation, yoga is much more than that and may be a valuable tool for achieving total health.

Yoga can also help with chakra unblocking, activation, and healing. Yoga practice provides us with insights that we would not be able to obtain in any other manner. This internal awareness is essential for recognizing each chakra both independently and as a linked entity, which aids us in understanding what is going on within our bodies.

Everyone may perform yoga, irrespective of age, gender, weight, or any other issue preventing them from doing so. While yoga might be more difficult for some, it is not the same for everyone. It is critical not to compare yourself to others when practicing yoga because your body will seem extremely different from your neighbor's physique. It is critical to recognize that adjustments can and should be made to accommodate your body. There is nothing wrong with adjusting a yoga position to meet your individual needs.

It's also worth noting that a well-balanced yoga practice incorporates both passive and energetic styles of yoga, which are sometimes referred to as yin and yang. Yoga poses that are more passive and restorative are equally as vital as those that are more dynamic and stimulating. I'll talk a lot about creating balance in this book, and this component of yoga is no exception. In contrast, the intensity of an aggressive yoga posture or program and a passive, vital part of the practice must also be included.

Consistent practice is the key to getting the most out of your yoga practice. Changes and effects will not occur overnight. Yoga may help you achieve many excellent things, including a better and happier life, but you will not experience results if you do not put in consistent effort.

Practicing the Essential Poses

This book contains thorough descriptions of yoga postures and sequences to assist you in connecting with and awakening your chakra-healing potential. I describe each posture and, if applicable, alteration possibilities straightforwardly. The yoga sequences are simple to follow and are particularly intended to help you on your path to a healthy and balanced mind and body.

In addition to the yoga asana instructions, there are other advice and activities to include in your yoga practice, such as breathing methods and meditation exercises. A healthy and well-rounded practice requires a blend of physical and mental yoga practices. Each yoga position, tip, and exercise are associated with a different chakra.

It is critical to learn which postures are closely related to each chakra so that you may tailor your yoga practice to your own needs. This book will walk you through every step of a chakra yoga practice. It will enable you to incorporate your own customized chakra yoga regimen into your daily life.

Practice Compassion

The key to reaching your health and wellbeing objectives is consistency in your yoga practice. Dedication, consistency, and focus will provide you with the results you're searching for.

While hard effort is essential for achieving objectives, it is equally critical to exercise self-compassion. It is just as vital to be kind to oneself to practice consistently. This implies that if you are unwell or unable to practice, you may continue your normal practice when you feel better. You may always change poses to fit your unique demands during your practice, from beginner to advanced. Never be humiliated or depressed if you need to adjust a pose — everyone's body is different.

Through a steady and well-rounded chakra yoga practice, you will be able to reach your health and wellness objectives over time if you have a combination of drive, focus, compassion, and patience.

Looking for Happiness

A balanced chakra feels renewed and invigorated, and you can sense energy moving smoothly through it inside your body. We are all aiming for this smooth flow of Prana, although it can be difficult to obtain. The flow of energy helps you to feel liberated both within and outside of your body. A free-flowing chakra provides you with a lot of energy and power in the region it is related to. It also delivers a balanced sense of serenity and quiet to that place.

A chakra that is obstructed frequently feels exactly that: blocked. It seems like the energy is trapped and sluggish, and it might hinder a full range of motion in that specific area of the body. A blocked chakra prevents the passage of Prana to the surrounding chakras from being balanced, producing issues in other regions. Depending on the chakra, it might cause your body to feel stiff in that area, or it can cause physical health concerns such as headaches, stomach discomfort, and joint pain. Depending on the chakra impact, it can also cause emotional or mental health difficulties such as anxiety, sadness, or phobias. These can be as debilitating as, if not more so than, physical diseases.

It takes time to see the effects of a focused chakra on yoga practice. You must pay attention to your body, commit to consistent practice, concentrate on the precise chakras and obstructed places, and require care.

It is necessary to care for the alignment of our chakras in the same way that we would go to the doctor for a yearly exam and look at our overall health. Even if you feel well and have no evident problems that require urgent treatment, taking care of your chakras and ensuring they remain balanced and aligned is critical to having a healthy and balanced life.

Peace and Healing

An overactive chakra indicates that too much energy is pouring into that area. A blockage might produce this in a nearby chakra, or it can be created by trauma to that location, which draws in additional energy to speed up the healing process. Although having extra energy appears to be a positive thing, it might damage more than good. An excess of energy in a particular chakra can also cause issues.

An underactive chakra does not have enough energy flowing to it. A blockage can cause a nearby chakra that prevents a significant quantity of the body's energy supply from reaching it. This causes the chakra to take on a more passive function in the body, and as a result, it is unable to act in tandem with the other chakras. In the afflicted region, this produces sluggishness and a lack of mobility.

A balanced chakra feels liberated, invigorated, energetic, and at peace. It contains just enough energy to keep that section of the body operating properly and communicating with the rest of the body. Our objective is to have a balanced chakra system as a whole.

Because the body and mind are so inextricably linked, it is vital to remember that achieving balance in one frequently leads to alleviation in the other. When an emotional or mental health issue is healed and balance is restored, we frequently discover that our corresponding physical issues subside or disappear entirely. Many people are surprised by this since there is a frequent assumption that the body and mind should be considered different. This couldn't be further from the truth and learning more about your chakras is an excellent way to see how.

A chakra yoga practice tailored to your specific requirements will help you attain chakra balance and general healing. This can give short-term pain relief while healing badly neglected emotional issues, allowing you to live a better life and feel better. A chakra yoga practice that balances your chakra system can also bring long-term advantages that can be observed in your health as you age.

CHAPTER 17: CHAKRAS TYPES, YOGA & MEDITATION

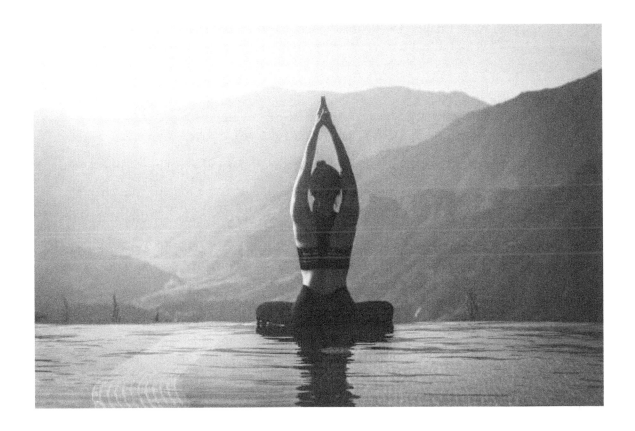

While some individuals say there are up to 114 different types of chakras, most people only consider the top seven. Each chakra is in charge of a distinct collection of moods, emotions, organs, and actions. They have their color and positioning on the bottom as well. We'll go further into the understanding of each of the seven chakras. We'll begin at the bottom of your spine, known as the "Root Chakra," and work our way up to the top of your spine, known as the "Crown Chakra." This sequence progresses from the first to the seventh chakra. You will learn all you need to know about each one along the road.

The Root Chakra

The Root Chakra is the first of the seven chakras. This brilliant red chakra is placed between your legs at the base of your spine. This chakra is connected with an earthy brown tone rather than a red one in certain books or teachings.

The Root Chakra is in charge of feeling anchored and steady in your life and secure. Anxiety is the most prevalent symptom that this chakra is misaligned. This symptom can occur whether this chakra is under or over-activated.

When your Root Chakra is underactive, you will feel insecure or fearful in your daily life. If it is hyperactive, you may feel trapped in your ways or find it difficult to accept transition or change in your life. The most effective approach to balance this chakra is to meditate and practice grounding practices. As a result, you will be able to ease many of the associated symptoms.

This chakra is linked to organs such as the kidney, reproductive glands and organs, and the spine. If you have problems with kidney infections or discomfort, difficulty reproducing or with reproductive hormones, or pain in your spinal column, your Root Chakra may be misaligned. You can restore chakra balance and alleviate stress in these systems.

Root Chakra – Meditation

- Find a comfortable position to lie or sit in.
- Focus your attention on your breath and begin softly breathing and expelling to boost your calm.
- Allow your mind to wander and allow your ideas to eventually come to your root chakra.
- Spend some time imagining what it will look like. Examine its color, size, health, and so on.
- Breathe air down to your root on your next inhalation. Feel this area of your body fill up with air. Continue to take deep breaths like this while you contemplate this chakra while you're here.
- Investigate any thoughts, pictures, or ideas that arise. Try not to avoid any strong emotions, suppressed memories, or ideas that arise.
- Continue to breathe for a few moments as you investigate anything that "happens here." Don't be frightened to let any deeper sentiments rise and come to the surface. Pay attention to your feelings and become conscious of them.
- Now, get ready to let go of this energy. When you let it all go, it may look any way you want it to when you use your inner eye to observe it. It may either explode out of you like a rocket or spill out like a torrent.
- As you take many deep inhales and exhales, visualize the discharge of harmful energy.
- As you release, say to yourself in your head or out loud, "I am comfortable in my strength and have all I need to survive." I am a grounded person that strives for steadiness in myself and my life. I let go of my worry, fears, and doubts that I don't have enough. I'm ready to let go of old scars, traumas, and challenges from this portion of myself. I am ready to let go of whatever fears I have about my past, present, or future. I'm a solid foundation. I am strong in my capacity to sink my roots into the ground and make my existence sturdy and secure. "I am my own home."
- As you say this or something similar, imagine your root chakra whirling around at a relaxing and slow pace, enabling its color to feel bright and strong and its vibrational frequency to fluctuate or rise.
- Refocus your attention on your entire body and resume normal breathing. Lie in this posture for as long as you need to unwind and digest your root chakra healing findings.

Based on how long you choose to dwell on your energy, this meditation might take a variety of lengths.

Root Chakra – Yoga

Crow Pose

1. Make sure your legs are three feet apart when you stand. Concentrate on your spine, which should be rising from your pelvis area. You will also notice an even distribution of your weight between your feet on the ground or land underneath you.

2. Squat gently while keeping your feet planted on the ground. Attach your hands in a prayer position and insert your elbows inside your two knees to assist you in maintaining a straight posture.

3. Inhale deeply and gently into your abdomen, hold your breath for several minutes, then exhale fully empty lungs. Repeat for another 20 to 30 minutes.

4. Let go of your hands and lie down for a few minutes. Allow the breath to flow naturally when you have released it. You will observe Prana circulating through your perineum and other adjacent areas of your body, particularly your coccyx and hips.

You will master this root chakra yoga with more practice, and it will make you feel pleased and worthy of your being.

The Sacral Chakra

The Sacral Chakra is the second of the seven chakras. This chakra is placed between the hips, above the pelvis. The color orange is associated with this chakra.

The Sacral Chakra governs your passion, sexuality, and creativity. When your Sacral Chakra is underactive, you may find it difficult to create, feel indifferent or inflexible, or cut off from intimacy. When this chakra is very underactive, you may feel a lack of closeness physically and emotionally. Alternatively, if this chakra is hyperactive, you may feel incredibly sexual, to the point that you are labeled a sex addict. You may also discover that you are prone to being emotionally involved quickly. In any case, you must take the time to balance your Sacral Chakra. You may do this through meditation, awareness, and the use of some of the natural approaches outlined later in this book.

This chakra is closely related to your gallbladder, adrenal glands, immune system, waste organs, metabolism, and spleen. When you have problems with any of these chakras, you should take the time to restore balance to your Sacral Chakra. You will most likely reduce a major portion of your undesirable side effects and symptoms.

Sacral Chakra – Meditation

- Begin this meditation in the same way you began the root chakra meditation. The bath is a perfect place to practice this meditation. This is the chakra related to water and connecting to water can offer another layer of connection to your chakra healing.

- Find a comfortable sitting or sleeping posture and reconnect with your breathing. With this chakra, you will want to go deeper into your emotions. Be prepared to cry, laugh, or express yourself if something comes up that has to be expressed.

- Spend a lot of time focusing on the orangey tone of your second chakra as you breathe in and out. Consider the energy to be a swirl of orange water whirling in your lower belly.

- Direct your attention to this place with your breath. Breathe into your sacral chakra and sense its liquid essence with each inhalation. For many minutes, maintain this breathing concentration and attention to the color and sensation of this chakra.

- What comes to mind when you look at the water at this location? Are there any people, locations, or items visible on the water's surface? Do you have any sensations, ideas, or thoughts concerning anything?

- As you breathe into this chakra, pay attention to your sensations. What do you hear going on around you? Is there anything you can smell? What do you have in your mind's eye? What are you touching that you can feel right now? Connect with the energy of the second chakra by using all five of your senses.

- Bring any problems to the surface of the orange water and visualize all of your problems, anxieties, repressed energy, and emotions. Consider a boat of some type approaching the water of your sacral chakra. Consider all the bad concerns or feelings making their way into the boat.

- Breathe down to this chakra with a deep, long, slow inhalation, and hold your breath for 10 seconds. Watch the boat sail away from your body and out of sight as you breathe.

- Say aloud or in your head the following: "I am full of pleasure, passion, and desire." I have a lot of creative and influential thoughts. I have the right to have feelings about people, places, and things. I am willing to connect with both myself and others. I am ready to let go of whatever barriers are keeping me from embracing my compassion, sensuality, sexuality, and the fruits of my creativity. I am an unlimited and limitless source of light and life. I am drawn to the energy of passionate production and lovely feeling. When it feels good for me to connect with others or be sensual and sexual with others, I will choose to do so. I am my power, and I will pick how to express myself most naturally. As a human with feelings and emotions, I accept my own needs. My difficulties, fears, aches, and concerns about my energy of passion, desire, sex, and creation are sent away on this boat. I have all the energy I need to live my life."

- You can edit the wording to represent the specific concerns arising for you at this moment. It is your responsibility to understand what your energy is telling you to let go of; therefore, be precise to yourself and your requirements. These are some examples of what you could say.

When you've done this phase of the meditation, focus on your breath and rest for a few minutes while you ponder.

Open your eyes and carry on with your day, feeling rejuvenated. It may be beneficial to journal what you saw in your vision or create a colorful representation of who you are or what you have released.

Sacral Chakra – Yoga

Pelvic Lifts

1. Lie down on the ground with your spine flat. As you face upwards, your head should also be on the ground. Feel your breath as it flows through your nose and into your lungs and pay attention to the movement of your rib cage as it rises and falls as you fill your lungs.

2. Bend your knees and point them straight up at the sky. Ascertain that your spirits are fully flat and near your spread arms on the ground. Your palms should also be touching the ground. Place your long middle finger on your ankles to keep in the proper position.

3. Slowly inhale and elevate your pelvis to the maximum height possible. Lift your spine slowly, starting with the lowest vertebrae. The spinal column should then be moved carefully.

4. Exhale as you gently return your spine to its previous position. As you return to your old posture on the ground, the vertebrae will rejoin.

5. For at least 20 minutes, repeat the motion of raising your pelvis up and down. Maintain a steady, smooth, calm, and contemplative movement. Your breath should direct the movement; make sure your lungs are full, your spine and arms are fully extended, and exhale as you go back down. Allow your spine to be in charge of moving the rest of your body. Also, imagine that your breath is erasing all of your stress. Perform 3 to 6 lifts.

6. Believe that all of the emotions you are experiencing are intended to heal and restore balance and harmony. If you practice this type of yoga, you will notice some improvements, and your sacral chakra will be properly repaired.

The Solar Plexus Chakra

The third chakra is the Solar Plexus Chakra, and its location may appear clear. It is placed right above the belly button, near the solar plexus. This golden yellow chakra is a strong one that is profoundly connected to many aspects of our existence.

The Solar Plexus Chakra governs sentiments of self-assurance, willpower, personal strength, and force. The emotional consequences of any imbalance inside the chakra will be tough to handle. With an underactive Solar Plexus Chakra, you will experience feelings of powerlessness, timidity, or lack of self-confidence. If you have poor self-esteem, it is related to this chakra. You may also be lacking in direction or purpose in your life. When this chakra is hyperactive, you may be potentially aggressive or dominating, striving to be the "boss" of situations. Either way, you should not strive for it. Bringing balance to this chakra can help you feel more confident and empowered without feeling the need to become overbearing.

The Solar Plexus Chakra is related to the upper spine, liver, stomach, pancreas, and metabolism. When this chakra is out of whack, you may suffer discomfort or illness in any of these systems. When you bring the chakras into balance, it is probable that they will work more effectively and that your general well-being will improve.

Solar Plexus – Meditation

- If you have access to sunlight, this is an excellent meditation.

- First, relax your body in a comfortable posture, such as sitting or lying down.

- Pay close attention to your breathing. To begin, take long, calm, deep breaths.

- Once you've connected with yourself in this position, take a deep breath of fire to activate your solar plexus energies. The fire breath consists of fast bursts of inhalation into the nose and exhalation through the nose, pulsating the belly (like panting with your mouth closed). Make sure your tummy moves in and out, and your diaphragm moves up and down.

- Practice the fire breath for a few rounds before returning to deep and relaxed inhales and exhales.

- Visualize your solar plexus as a sunny golden color. As you watch the energy whirl in this place, bring your breath into it. You might imagine your solar plexus as a little sun if you wish.

- Give yourself some time to work on this vision. Take note of any thoughts, ideas, or sensations that arise while you spend time here. They may not always be precisely what you expect, especially chakra attributes. You may consider your boss or your relationship. Images of an altercation you had with a grocery clerk may appear in your mind. Anything that comes up here has to deal with this energy, and while you focus on it, think about how this chakra has been engaged with people, places, or things. (For example, thinking about your boss when clearing this chakra might refer to wanting to be the boss one day but not feeling sufficient, or having a problem with how your boss makes you feel like you don't know what you're doing or talking about, etc.)

- Feel these energies arise, and as you honor and acknowledge to yourself what they may signify, bring greater attention to boosting the brilliance of light emanating from this chakra.

- Allow whatever energies to have arisen to be healed and purified to be brought into the light of this chakra. See the sun's scorching heat setting fire to these energies to cleanse and liberate them. Allow the light of yourself to spark your strength and let go of whatever negative notions you may have about yourself here.

- As you burn away these energy, thoughts, and ideas, say or think something like this: "I am my power, and I allow myself to take up space in this world as myself. Right now, I can see who I am clearly. I am a person of honesty, integrity, and drive, and I have my aspirations. I act on the things that allow me to be my most authentic self. I have all the energy and health I need to propel my development. I'm fine with making errors since I'll learn from them and improve. I know exactly what I want and how long it will take me to get there. My path always involves other people, and it is always OK for me to be myself in their presence. I am not frightened to take action in the direction that my life requires."

- When you feel like you've acquired a degree of self-confidence with your ideas and words, see your inner sun beaming brilliantly as you take in a few more rounds of deep, long inhales and exhales.

- After a few cycles, open your eyes and repeat the fire breath. Continue your day feeling strong and self-assured.

Solar Plexus – Yoga

Front Platform

1. Lie down on your stomach, with your toes pointed in the other direction or away from your head. Bend your elbows and place your palms on the ground.

2. Inhale and lift your torso upwards as if performing a press-up but keep your toes facing the opposite or backward.

3. Hold that upward posture for a few seconds, then take a deep inhale and suck it into your abdomen, followed by lengthy exhales as you push your air out. Spend at least three minutes focusing on and experiencing the Prana flowing through the navel core.

This yoga practice will aid in the healing and balance of your Solar Plexus Chakra.

The Heart Chakra

The Heart Chakra is the fourth of the seven chakras. This chakra is related to the color green and is situated just behind your rib cage. As you might expect, it is placed right next to your heart. This chakra is also known as the "Heart Center" by others. The literature on energy healing and the energy body appears to be used interchangeably. In this book, we'll refer to it as the Heart Chakra.

The Heart Chakra is in charge of sentiments of love and compassion. When your Heart Chakra is underactive, you may find it difficult to feel love or compassion for the people and things in your life. You may even find it difficult to feel these emotions for yourself. If your Heart Chakra is hyperactive, you may find yourself loving and giving compassion so freely that you become attached or overly sympathetic towards others. If one of these conditions occurs, you must balance your Heart Chakra. You may do so by going within and determining what is driving you to be one way or the other. Emotional experiences in our life can often drive us to be exceedingly frigid or extremely loving towards others.

This chakra is associated with the heart, lungs, and thymus gland. If you are experiencing problems with either of these, you may want to undertake some energy balancing work with your heart chakra to restore balance and harmony. This may provide relief from any sickness that is bothering you.

Heart Chakra – Meditation

- As with sacral meditation, this meditation will expand your heart chakra, and you may experience deep and powerful sensations. Allow your emotions to come to you. Try not to suppress whatever you are thinking or feeling. We carry a lot of sorrow and trauma in our hearts, and even when we think we're doing well in this area, there's always something deep down that needs some love and attention.

- Sit comfortably in a chair or on the floor in a lotus stance.

- Pay attention to your breathing. Deeply inhale and exhale several times to center yourself and connect to your meditation.

- Take a deep breath into your heart and feel its vitality. Consider the emerald green hue and how it feels. Big? Small? Quiet? Tight? Expansive?

- Keep breathing into this space and exploring the energy of the heart chakra. What visuals are appearing? What are your opinions and ideas? Do you already have an abundance of love in your life? Do you think you love yourself enough?

- Spend time with these thoughts and sensations as you grow closer to opening up to them. Is there one that keeps coming up? If this is the case, the concept, picture, or feeling wishes for you to spend some time contemplating it. Where will it lead you? When you follow that emotion, what or who do you see? How does it make you feel?

- Connect to these realities by meditating on each section of your heart, requesting that you connect to the knowledge. As you look, you may sense a shift in your energy. You may feel like sobbing aloud, followed by a sensation of inner serenity and tranquility after releasing yourself.

- Bring your hands to your heart and rest them palms down on the middle of your chest. You breathe into your palms and experience this chakra's green light and energy.

- With your hands over your heart, silently or aloud recite these words or something similar: "I am love. I am entitled to love and be loved. I am capable of giving and receiving love from others and myself. I choose to cultivate a loving attitude in my life by accepting all individuals and all of my interactions with them. I am working on self-awareness via love. I am linked to my heart as a sensitive, compassionate, and responsive person. I'd like to learn how to operate with loving energy in my life. I let go of any prior pains concerning my heart that have kept me locked off here. I realize it's okay to guard myself and my emotions against getting wounded, but I'm also open-hearted. I will connect more deeply via my heart and sentiments as I go through life. I am ready to love myself and others."

- After saying or thinking these phrases, return your attention to your breath for a few seconds. When you're ready to end your meditation, take your hands away from your heart and wrap your arms around your body in an embrace. Hold yourself for as long as you want and truly allow yourself to feel held (at least a few minutes). Continue to breathe deeply as you wrap your arms around yourself.

- Relax your arms and allow a grin to grow on your lips. Carry on with your day as planned.

Heart Chakra – Yoga

Heart-Centering Meditation

1. Kneel and take a seat on your heels. Maintain a straight posture with your spine. As the diaphragm and solar plexus are elevated slightly, feel the flow of your breath as it enters your lungs.

2. Connect your middle fingers while stretching your elbows sideways like flying wings, keeping your forearms parallel to the ground.

3. Lower your eyelids or close your eyes halfway and concentrate on the tip of your nose. Other styles of yoga employ the eye position to focus, cleanse, calm the mind, and activate the pineal and pituitary glands.

4. In your head, you will hear a vibrating inner voice repeating the mantra "Humme Hum Bram hum." While doing this sort of yoga, you can also listen to a recorded version of this mantra.

5. As you listen to this phrase, slowly extend your hands out. Slowly inhale and exhale, feeling the Prana flow from the core of your heart and spreading throughout your entire body.

The Throat Chakra

As you might expect, the fifth chakra, known as the Throat Chakra, is located within the throat. The color associated with this chakra is a vivid and brilliant blue. It is typically portrayed as a light blue hue, although it may be represented as any shade of blue.

This chakra is in charge of open communication and self-expression. When this chakra is underactive, you may feel withdrawn or frustrated, grief, or rage because you are not speaking your truth. If it is hyperactive, you may speak excessively and fail to filter yourself to the point perceived as domineering or impolite. Or you may be a lousy listener who only listens for the chance to respond. When you have either of these symptoms, you must build a mindfulness practice and enable yourself to recover control of your voice. Suppose you feel as if you are hiding your truth. In that case, you should work on being honest, or you should work on keeping ideas to yourself or learning to censor yourself if you are offering information or opinions too freely to the point that it is impeding your life.

The Throat Chakra is linked to the respiratory system, thyroid, and other organs related to the throat and mouth. If you have any problems with these organs, you may be suffering from physical signs of an imbalanced chakra. The most often reported symptom is the sensation of a lump in the throat. You may remove or alleviate these symptoms by restoring balance to your throat chakra and speaking your truth without speaking too loudly.

Throat Chakra – Meditation

- You can start this meditation in a chair, on the floor, or lying on your back.
- Get into a comfortable posture and concentrate on your breathing. Allow yourself to get grounded and comfortable by connecting with your body.
- Because the throat wants to create noise, you should plan to be in a place where it is OK to be loud or verbally expressive.
- Maintain your breathing by using the alternate nostril breath method you learned. Try a few rounds of this to get your breathing technique more closely related to your upper body.
- If you're sitting, attempt a few neck rolls and stretches to open up your neck energy.
- Concentrate on your breathing and keep it calm and deep.

- Press your tongue on the roof of your mouth. And then take a long, deep breath through your nose. Begin to exhale by invoking an "L" sound, as if you were going to say "La." Inhale for three breath cycles, then exhale with this sound intoned. Try to hold the noises for as long as you can with your breath.

- Make a humming sound while following the same breathing directions as step 7. Begin by intoning "hum," and when you shut your mouth to produce the "M," keep your lips together so you can feel them vibrating. Maintain a relaxed mouth. This intonation should be repeated three times during your inhales and exhales.

- After that, make a "Ha" sound. Allow your tongue and jaw to relax and drop as you open your mouth to let the "Ha" come out on the exhale. Rep three times more.

- Visualize the light of this chakra vibrating and rippling with the sound of your voice as you intone. Allow this blue hue to fill your throat, lungs, and mouth as you expel these noises. Imagine your breath exiting your body as the same hue as your throat chakra if you choose.

- Pay attention to how you feel when making these noises. Are you self-conscious? Are you remaining quiet but wishing you could be louder? Do you get a scratchy or raspy feeling in this area? Are there any thoughts or ideas that come to mind concerning people, places, or things that need to be focused on?

- When creating these noises, allow yourself to invent sounds and finish the L, Hum, Ha cycles. Make whatever noise that seems natural to you or as though it has to be expelled. Allow yourself to enjoy it. Try not to have any say over what comes out.

- Pay attention to your energies in this situation. Are you attempting to exert control over the sounds emanating from your body? Do you recognize your voice, or does it sound strange to you?

- When you've created these noises, relax and restore your attention to your breathing. To keep your throat chakra activated and open, repeat the following affirmations aloud: "I have my voice, and I want to be heard." It's OK if I have anything to say. I am just as open to hearing other people's words as I am to hearing my own. I communicate well. I can communicate the truth about myself and my knowledge. I am a strong vibrational and acoustic instrument. I'd like to express myself honestly through my ideas, feelings, and words. I have the right to speak freely, just as I have the right not to speak when I don't want to. "I am capable of comprehending my truthful statements."

- Feel free to change the wording to match your personal experience with chakra energy. Continue to take deep breaths for several minutes before going on with your day.

Throat Chakra – Yoga

Camel

1. Kneel on the floor, keeping your legs apart. Place your palms on your ankles gently as you lean back in the same posture.
2. Breathe in and let your heart rise as your thighs and hips push forward.

3. Draw your shoulders towards each other while breathing to allow your heart to expand more profoundly. Put your hands on your back to help you exhale more easily.

4. Concentrate on your neck while deeply inhaling. Keep pushing your hips forward to allow the sternum to expand.

5. Return your head to its normal posture and gently place your hands on your ankle.

6. Relax and let Prana heal your throat as it generates a subtle internal vibrating sound "hmm" Continue for at least three minutes or longer after releasing the sound.

This chakra's successful performance will enable you to make aware decisions and transmit real expressions that emerge from our true sense.

The Third Eye Chakra

The Third Eye Chakra is situated between and slightly above your brows. This chakra is represented by the color indigo and is the sixth of the seven chakras. For many, this is the most well-known chakra, as it is mentioned in literature and spiritual teachings.

The Third Eye Chakra is in charge of connecting you to your intuition, psychic vision, and insight. When you have an underactive chakra, you may find it difficult to connect with your intuitive side or feel lost and wandering through life. Alternatively, if it is hyperactive, you may become anxious about your gut impulses and overanalyze little events in your life. You should meditate to balance this chakra. Whether the chakra is underactive or hyperactive, your meditation might aim to calm it or open it up. Consequently, it should return you to a healthy flow in which you can acknowledge and listen to your intuition without developing anxiety or paranoia about the information it provides.

The Third Eye Chakra is physically linked to your pineal gland, pituitary gland, eyes, hormones, and brain. If you have a misalignment in this chakra, you might have various problems with either of these organs. You may suffer headaches behind your eyes or visual problems; you may endure regular headaches or "brain fog," hormonal changes that impair your wellness, or hyperactive or underactive pineal and pituitary glands. Bringing this chakra back into balance should help you treat various diseases.

Third Eye Chakra – Meditation

- There are several methods to connect to the source of your higher vision and intuition. This is a simple type of meditation, but as you progress in chakra work, you may instinctively change it to be more fit for your current requirements.

- Lie down on the floor or in a quiet spot where you will not be disturbed. Relax here and concentrate on your breathing.

- Concentrate on your breathing for many minutes. Some individuals will be told where to go by their Third Eye and will be able to continue a meditation instinctively from this point.

- If you are not naturally directed by your "seeing," you may work on becoming more in tune with that energy here. Consider your brow chakra. Look at the color indigo.

- Close your eyes and move them to "look" at the location in your mind where your Third Eye is (up and inward).

- Spend some time with your deep inhales and exhales while your eyes are concentrated like this under closed eyelids. Continue to visualize your chakra's brightness and color.

- As you gaze at this energy, notice how it begins to extend, like a rod or shaft protruding from your brow. Extend it as far as possible. It can travel to the roof of your room, house, or apartment building, the clouds, or the universe.

- What do you perceive as you connect with this vision? What are your plans? Pay close attention to the particulars. Outside of yourself, feel the energy of this connection. If your eyes get tired of staring up and in, you can rest them.

- Once your Third Eye energy has been expanded up and out of you, relax into your breath and pay attention to any visuals that arise. You may also have ideas and sensations, which are frequently accompanied by imagery.

- Allow your thoughts to think on this while going on your "inner trip."

- Stay in this area for as long as you need to till the photographs are finished. Back down in your forehead, connect with your Third Eye energy, and repeat in your thoughts the following words, or something similar: "I can see more than what is in front of my face and eyes. I can see beyond what is seen on Earth. I am endowed with enormous insight and the ability to delve far into the big unknown. My vision goes beyond what is ordinarily seen, and I am proud of my openness to the spirit and the unknown. I am not terrified of this gift and look forward to utilizing it regularly. My soul is old and intelligent, and I am ready to release any prior experiences that have kept me from connecting to this reality. I am thankful for my ability to see."

- Take some time here to contemplate and breathe. You may fall asleep in this state, which is OK. When dealing with this chakra, it is usual.

- Take pleasure in the repercussions of this encounter while you go about your regular activities.

Third Eye Chakra – Yoga

Guru Namaste

1. Sit on your heels and in an erect stance to begin this yoga practice. Inhale deeply and notice how Prana enters your body with each breath. Try a firm cushion or blankets if you have trouble sitting on your heels.

2. Extend your arms towards the ground while spreading your knees comfortably. Maintain your spine's elongation by resting your forehead on the ground ahead and moving your lower back.

3. Concentrate on the spine between the shoulders to allow the heart to expand by melting that region.

4. As you inhale and exhale deeply, clasp your palms together and picture light. Also, relax and let gravity take over. Perform this yoga for at least 5 minutes.

5. Place your arms on the ground and slowly raise your torso, beginning with the lowermost spine and working your way up vertebrae by vertebra, finishing with raising your head. Take a few minutes to relax or lie on your back before rising.

You will notice a difference after doing this style of yoga and learn that you can easily utilize reasoning and make good judgments.

The Crown Chakra

The color purple corresponds to your Crown Chakra, which is located on top of your scalp at your head. However, other people think that this chakra is associated with the color white. You can use whichever one speaks to you, but we'll go with purple for this book and these lectures. This chakra is regarded as the seventh of seven chakras.

The Crown Chakra is in charge of providing individuals with wisdom, being in sync with the cosmos, and connecting them to the spiritual realm. When this chakra is inactive, you may feel distant from your spirit and as if you are making a series of rash judgments. When hyperactive, you may feel your head is in the clouds, and you cannot connect with reality. Because none of these are desirable symptoms, you must restore balance to the chakra to treat them. When it is working properly, you will be able to maintain a healthy connection to the spiritual realm while being securely anchored in your life. If you have an overactive chakra, you should ground yourself to bring yourself back down to Earth. If it is dormant, you should meditate and make the intention to reactivate your capacity to engage with the spiritual realm.

This chakra is in charge of the brain, the pineal gland, your biological cycles, and your spinal cord. When it is out of balance, you may feel any of these symptoms. Your pineal gland may not operate properly; you may struggle to sleep well or excessively; you may suffer pain in your lumbar area, "brain fog," or frequent headaches. If you are experiencing a number of these symptoms, or if one of them is persistent and difficult to manage, you may want to explore healing and balance your Crown Chakra. It might be imbalanced and cause a lack of happiness in these areas.

When you look at a chakra map, you may observe that the colors of the rainbow are synchronized. This information is useful since it will help you recall which hue corresponds to the chakra. Remember that red is at the bottom and purple is at the top. Each chakra is connected with its color, feelings, habits, and organs. When one is underactive, hyperactive, or otherwise misaligned, you may have symptoms related to everything your chakra is in charge of. If you are suffering specific symptoms, you may wish to revisit the chakras to discover which one corresponds to the location of your symptoms. Then you may work with that chakra to bring it into balance and harmony, potentially alleviating some or all of your problems.

Crown Chakra – Meditation

- Begin this meditation sitting on the floor or in a chair. Begin with your breath to anchor yourself in your practice.

- As you concentrate on your breathing, ground your root energy to where you are seated. Assume you have roots growing from your root and into the floor and dirt beneath your area.

- As you take calm, soothing breaths, see your entire chakra system waking up and coming to life. Visualize energy flowing freely throughout your entire body.

- While visualizing this energetic flow through all chakras, clasp your hand's palm to palm and place them in front of your heart chakra.

- Continue to breathe in and out as you feel your energy flow through all six chakras, and when you reach the seventh chakra at your crown, see the light of your being shoot out of the top of your head, like a bright rainbow.

- Allow this rainbow of light to be a continuous shaft of energy connecting you to the universe. Feel its link to the galaxy and everything that is beyond.

- Visualize your tree roots anchoring you to the earth as you breathe while the rainbow of light streaming from your crown connects you to the heavens.

- Keep this image in your Third Eye while saying or thinking the following phrases or something similar: "I am a synthesis of all energy. I am composed of light and vibration, and I am here to become more in sync with everything around me. I am a source of good life-force energy, and my totality witnesses the entire Universe. I'm letting go of whatever worries, concerns, or thoughts I've had throughout my life that I'm not one with everything and everyone. I am ready to let go of whatever grief and suffering have kept me from realizing my unlimited essence. I am prepared to travel my life path with purpose and the energy I know as my entire self. I believe that I am here for a reason and that every one of us has a distinct and vital mission. I am alive to the creative force."

- Visualize whatever concerns you have about your energy potential flowing out of the rainbow light from your head and into the universe for a change. Accept your life force as you pull your hands down from your heart.

- Place your hands, palms up, on your knees, and breathe in this position for a few moments. Relax and appreciate the feeling of being anchored to Earth and linked to the universe around you.

- Hold this stance for as long as you need to before moving on to other things.

Crown Chakra – Yoga

Guru Prasad's

1. Sit on your heels and let the light fill your spinal column as you ascend the column. Take a few deep breaths and notice how the Prana travels through your body.

2. Make a bowl-shaped structure with your hands, then position your palms facing the sky in front of your heart. The bowl's function is to collect unseen light.

3. Put your upper arms up against your rib cage. Feel the universe's treasures being poured into your hands. The presents will arrive one after the other, just as the favors have. As you perform this yoga, feel the presence of the limitless cosmos.

4. Concentrate on your nose tip and lower eyelid, leaving only a little hole in your eyes. The focus will assist you in opening your Third Eye, and the pineal gland will also stimulate your optic nerve. However, as you continue to meditate, you are free to close your eyes to focus more on your Third Eye.

5. Take long, deep breaths and exhale completely while allowing the feelings of love and compassion to enter your heart.

6. Also, open yourself up to accept benefits in various forms, such as consciousness and the boundless cosmos.

7. For at least 3 minutes, practice this type of meditation. You can take additional time if you believe you need it to repair your head chakra thoroughly.

If we allow the free flow of Prana and repair our head chakra, our awareness will flourish.

Yoga Pose Malasana

Squat with your palms together, take a deep breath, hold for 30 seconds, and then exhale easily. Tuck your toes into your feet and put your torso on your knees as you perform this yoga posture. Lifting your toes to pull them out of the ground will break your connection with the earth. This posture will help you connect with the earth, and the earth's energy is felt via the feet as you practice.

Uttanasana

Stand up and fold your arms together, contacting your right elbow with your left palm and your left hand to your left elbow. Rest your folded hands on your head crown, then lean and bow forward at the waist, arms and hands remaining folded. Relax your thoughts by doing this yoga. This will allow us to regain our calm and focus. It also relieves stiffness across our entire back.

The Mountain Pose

It is a chakra yoga practice that stands erect like a tree and experiences the earth's support. This position helps us feel grounded by allowing us to focus on the present moment. Also, do this yoga on the ground or grass to help you connect with the earth more deeply.

Salutations to the Sun

It also resembles a cobra serpent's posture. Lie face down on the ground with your stomach. Lift your upper body (from the waist up while still lying down) and face the sun with your palm hands. Slowly inhale and exhale, and you will begin to feel more connected, more powerful, and heat rising throughout your body. You have the option of closing or opening your eyes.

Anjaneyasana

Stretch your quadriceps and psoas muscles in this stance. Its association with the chakras makes sense because it is linked to the fight-or-flight response. It is also linked to the first or Root Chakra. Inhale and exhale five times to give your muscles more time to transform residual flight or fight energy into a calm yet fearless inner strength.

Warrior 2

Pose like a warrior, with your hands stretched outside, one leg stretched, and the other slightly bent, as the name suggests. The position allows you to tap into your inner power and resolve.

The Bridge Pose

Lie flat on the ground and elevate your body with your upper back, supporting your stance with the soles of your feet firmly against the ground. This position will stimulate your throat chakra while also assisting your root chakra in releasing excess energy. This posture may also balance your Sacral, Solar Plexus, and Heart Chakras.

Broad-Legged Forward Fold

Stretch your legs and drop your head to meet the ground, using your hands to support yourself. This position will stretch the muscles in your lower back and groin. This gives your Root Chakra a chance to discharge energy into your body.

Savasana

Lie down with your back to the earth, facing upwards, to enable the earth to support your entire body. With each breathing cycle, inhale and exhale easily while repeating the phrases, "I am safe; I am supported." When we approach life from a grounded viewpoint, we tend to be more tranquil and cheerful, and this position allows us to accomplish just that while also strengthening ourselves.

CHAPTER 18: CHAKRAS BALANCING & HEALING

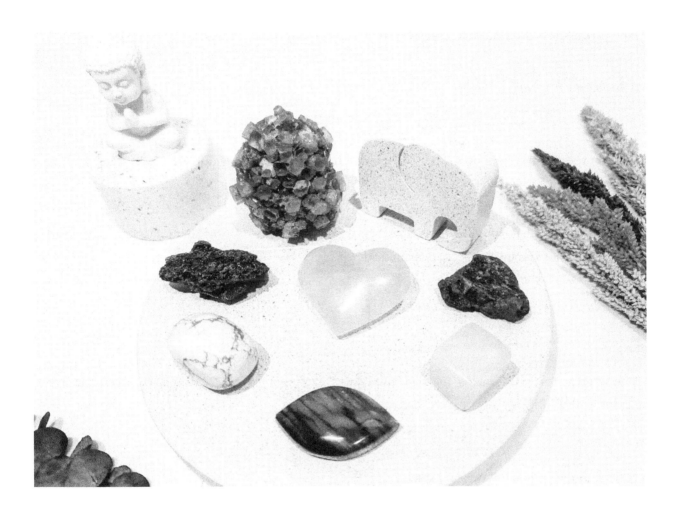

The Chakras and Crystal Healing

Crystals can be used for healing, ornamental jewelry, boost energy in an area, or as an elixir. Like everything else in the world, crystals are made up of vibrations. Every crystal has its unique vibration and energy.

When utilized for healing, the crystal stimulates the subtle energy system, aura, and chakras. Placing crystals on the chakras accelerates the healing process. Crystals can also be utilized as a stand-alone therapy or as part of a reiki session. They will boost any therapist's healing skill, making the healing session more potent.

Sometimes a crystal will refuse to work with a healer, a person, or when worn as part of a piece of jewelry. If this happens to you, you will be aware. Something will not feel quite right when worn as jewelry. It's possible that the crystal is too powerful for you at that moment or that the vibrations aren't perfect for you. The crystal must complement your vibes.

Some crystals vibrate slowly, whereas others vibrate significantly quicker. The more sensitive you are to energy, the more delicate vibrations you will pick up on from the stones. I've selected just two crystals that can be utilized to help repair each of the main chakras. There are many more, but I don't want to confuse or overwhelm you if you're just starting. Furthermore, the skill to operate with a few stones on each of the chakras to increase the healing process is more vital than understanding or using hundreds of crystals.

Ruby or Jasper for the Root Chakra

Ruby

It helps the reproductive system by re-energizing it and balancing blood sugar levels.

Jasper

Because this stone helps balance all chakras, it may be utilized to balance any of them. Jasper is particularly good for patients suffering from liver, spleen, or pancreatic issues.

Moonstone and Amber for the Sacral Chakra

Moonstone

This stone is great for harmonizing the digestive system, removing toxins (particularly from the liver), and helping ladies with PMS.

Amber

It is beneficial to the stomach, liver, and spleen.

Yellow Topaz and Citrine for the Solar Plexus Chakra

Yellow Topaz

It helps the neurological system, endocrine system, liver, and gallbladder.

Citrine

It aids in relaxation and calmness, as well as nervous system support.

Rose Quartz and Green Jade for the Heart Chakra

Rose Quartz

This stone aids in the emotional body's support and discharges feelings of hurt, rage, and other unpleasant emotions. It aids in the promotion of sentiments of tranquility.

Green Jade

Aids in emotional discharge and healing.

Aquamarine and Lapis Lazuli for the Throat Chakra

Aquamarine

This is a good stone for persons who regularly suffer from thyroid issues and sore throats. It is excellent for encouraging self-expression and aiding in reducing tension and anxiety.

Lapis Lazuli

This stone encourages peace and self-awareness. It aids in reducing stress and the maintenance of the immune system.

Indigo Sapphire and Turquoise for the Third Eye or Brow Chakra

Indigo Sapphire

This aids in promoting psychic awareness and removing bad energy from the aura and energy system.

Turquoise

This stone supports the immune system, alleviates sadness, and protects against psychic attacks.

Clear Quartz and Amethyst for the Crown Chakra

Clear Quartz

This stone can aid in the balance of all chakras. When applied to the Crown Chakra, it aids in the removal of bad energy and enhances a person's psychic powers.

Amethyst

This stone aids a person's spiritual journey. It aids in the removal of bad emotions and the reduction of headaches. Clear quartz stones: Place little clear quartz stones on all chakras to promote and intensify the healing process of the other stones.

How to Perform Chakra Healing Treatments

Preparation

- Make sure you have a calm, healing environment.
- If you have access to a therapeutic couch, it is preferable over a bed or anything like that. A couch is a better alternative because you won't have to bend and stretch as much as you would with a bed. Using a sofa might help you avoid injuries.
- Remove any heavy jewelry, belts, or shoes and lie on their back.
- Begin placing the crystals on the chakras while lying on the bed.
- Begin with the crown chakra, then move to the Third Eye, throat, heart, solar plexus, sacral, and base chakras.

Time Spent on Treatment

1. Leave for 15 minutes for the first session, progressively increasing to 30 minutes and never exceeding 60 minutes. Please remember that it should not be replaced if a crystal falls off. This is because the crystal may be too powerful for you, or it may not choose to work with that individual at that moment. You might try utilizing that specific crystal during the next session.
2. When the session is finished, remove the crystals in the sequence they were placed.
3. Place your hands a few inches above the head on the right side of the torso. Sweep outwards, following the body's curves down to the feet.
4. Repeat in the middle of the body and then on the left side.
5. You've just aided with the smoothing of the energy field.

Chakra Balancing and Blocking

When your chakras get blocked, the movement of energy into and out of your system and other chakras is hampered. This might have a detrimental impact on your overall well-being. Blocked chakras are often associated with certain psychological disorders and existential prejudices. Such existential prejudices limit your self-awareness in a variety of ways. You must open your chakras to recover emotionally and spiritually, as well as to avoid physical ailments. Energy healing may aid in the opening of your chakras and the restoration of your health.

First Chakra Blocked

When your first chakra is blocked, you worry about survival and security. You grow disoriented and begin to believe that you do not belong anyplace. You lack ideas and dreams, and your constitution begins to deteriorate.

You begin to grind and become excessively pragmatic. You also have difficulty letting go, and you have issues with your weight, colon, feet, bones, and legs.

Second Chakra Blocked

When your second chakra is obstructed, your vitality and libido suffer. You become emotionally detached and have difficulty dealing with change and enjoying enjoyment. You begin to hold back or become too emotional, sexual, and preoccupied with physical pleasure. You also begin to experience issues with your urinary and reproductive systems.

Third Chakra Blocked

You lack confidence and self-esteem when your third chakra is obstructed. You're having trouble visualizing your desires. You also abuse your authority and exercise domination over others. You also have tiredness, gastrointestinal issues, hypertension, diabetes, and allergies.

Fourth Chakra Blocked

Loneliness, difficulties giving or accepting love, a lack of emotional fulfillment, and a lack of compassion are all symptoms of a blocked fourth chakra. You also tend to remain in toxic partnerships. Love manifests at low frequencies when the fourth chakra is blocked. You also don't feel connected to nature or the Divine.

Fifth Chakra Blocked

When your fifth chakra is blocked, you find it difficult to communicate, express yourself, and share ideas with others. You begin to experience difficulties with your inventiveness. You start manipulating and deceiving yourself or others. You also have issues with your shoulders, neck, and thyroid.

Sixth Chakra Blocked

You lack inspiration, vision, and attention when your sixth chakra is blocked. Your intuition becomes confused, and you struggle to perceive the broader picture. You also develop skewed vision and imagination, delusions, and an overreliance on intellect and reasoning. You also begin to have visual issues and nightmares, and headaches.

Seventh Chakra Blocked

You become ungrounded, spacy, indecisive, and unrealistic when you have a blockage in your seventh chakra. You struggle to complete chores and feel unhappy, confused, and alienated. You also begin to have a sense of meaninglessness. You also increase your chances of developing mental illnesses and having difficulties with your brain and cognition.

Do You Need Chakra Balancing?

Your chakras are conduits for energy. It circulates up and down your core channel, spine, and head, connecting your chakras. It also moves horizontally, sharing energy with the rest of the cosmos.

When a chakra system is balanced, the following symptoms appear:

- All of the chakras get energy vertically. There isn't a single chakra that is obstructed.
- Energy travels horizontally, with each chakra exchanging energy with the rest of the universe.
- There isn't a single chakra that rotates slower or faster than the others. None of them are exceptionally inactive or hyperactive.
- All chakras are open to the extent required to promote your spiritual development and wellness. None of them are either tightly or too widely closed.
- Neither the lower nor upper chakras are too stressed.

Most energy healers can identify if the chakras are open, healthy, and balanced. However, it is not required to sense them to analyze and determine their balance condition. If your chakra system is out of harmony, it will show up in your thoughts, emotions, and life. When you have a healthy and balanced chakra system, you will notice the following:

- A healthy physique helps you on your spiritual path and gives your life meaning.
- You feel safe, grounded, confident, and in touch with your body.
- You are aware of your feelings and are not overwhelmed.
- You are at ease with your sexuality.
- You are self-assured and capable of expressing your dreams without the need to control others.
- You have connections that are healthy, caring, and compassionate.
- You can convey your truth.
- You have a strong sense of intuition.
- You have a deep sense of spiritual connectedness.

Methods for Chakra Balancing

There are two methods for balancing your chakras that are recommended:

Chakra Singing Bowl Balancer

You should meditate for a few minutes every morning. Then, using this technique, you should begin to balance and align your chakras. Start with the first chakra and work your way up. Hold your awareness of your first chakra and let its sound echo as your singing bowl vibrates. After a few minutes, sound your singing bowl for the second chakra, and so on. Continue repeating this until you are done with all your chakras.

Hands-On Chakra Balancer

It is a traditional approach for chakra balance. It is quite simple to accomplish. Begin by lying down on the ground. Ideally, you should be in a quiet place where no one can bother you. Breathe through your stomach and spend several minutes grounding and centering yourself. Try to align and balance your chakras. Place your palm on your first chakra or right above your groin. Place the other hand on the second chakra. Continue to place your hands on these points until you sense an energy equalization. Hold this pose for one to two minutes before moving on to the next chakra. Repeat the balancing process for each chakra. Get back up when you're finished. Drink a glass of water and go about your business.

Chakra Cleansing Meditation

You may purify your chakras using a variety of meditation practices. Our chakras may get clogged with bad or unneeded ideas and feelings, and if not cleared, they can spiral out of control, leading to diseases, sadness, and addictive habits such as drugs and alcoholism. You will also be unable to be productive or effective in anything you attempt to do. You must take the necessary measures and practice any procedures to purify your chakras to live a healthy and productive life.

Example of Chakra Cleansing Meditation

1. Sit comfortably on a flat surface or the ground. Inhale deeply and exhale slowly. Relax while performing the practice and connecting with the surroundings.
2. Listen carefully to noises inside you; these sounds might result from chakra cleansing.
3. Release anything you don't need, toss everything into the dirt, and be mindful of your surroundings and the rising and falling of your breath.
4. Breathe down to your roots and allow them to connect to the ground. Allow your root chakra to take all it requires and place it in your imagination.
5. Allow the energy to flow to your sacral chakra, breathe deeply, and exhale gently and calmly. Continue to your other chakras, including the Solar Plexus, Throat, Heart, Third Eye, and Crown. Allow enough time for these chakras to properly cleanse themselves and get rid of everything they don't need.

Continue with this cleansing meditation for at least 20 minutes, stopping only when you feel your chakras are completely cleansed.

Meditation on Heart Cleansing and Forgiveness

1. Begin by sitting with your back straight and softly inhaling and exhaling. Concentrate on the present moment.
2. Check if your consciousness is filled with a genuine desire to cleanse. Use the affirmation listed below.
3. "My genuine self reveals the truth about who I am."

4. Allow yourself to rid yourself of all unpleasant ideas and sensations. Be loyal to all of your feelings and let go of those you don't need.

5. Consider any individual or persons you may have had unfavorable thoughts towards, and it's best to start with those you have the most resentment for.

6. Invite your imagination to explain why you are resentful of a certain individual or group of people. If he is your employer, it might be due to their "controlling character." It might also be due to the "abusive temperament" of a coworker you dislike. Don't pass judgment on them; instead, consider whether you have similar tendencies.

7. Consider how you felt abused in the past.

8. Pretend the person who offends or mistreats you is in the room with you, and picture them saying or annoying you as they typically do while observing them. Allow them to stay in your fantasies until you feel their actions or statements no longer influence you.

9. You must understand that you are only words and bad habits, no matter how much they mistreat and abuse you, and look beyond and purify these beliefs.

This type of cleaning meditation should take at least 5 minutes.

You will be able to be less concerned by individuals you despise, and no matter how they continue to treat you, you will treat them with compassion without harboring any grudges or unpleasant thoughts towards them.

Sunlight Purification Cleansing Technique

1. This necessitates that you execute on a sunny day or during the day. The light acts as a reminder of your pure consciousness. Step outdoors, take a stance, and raise your hands.

2. Allow sunlight to enter your crown head and disseminate it to the rest of your body. Consider the brilliant sunshine purifying your chakras as it floods through the sites of the bodily parts that symbolize all seven chakras.

3. Also, envision this light flowing incessantly, and the washing is done fully and indefinitely.

4. Feel the chakras being nourished by pleasant ideas. Feel the heart chakra, for example, being flooded with pure love. Your throat was full of expressiveness and communicating capacity.

5. Imagine and feel the light purifying all of your body's organs, tissues, and muscles from one section of one chakra position to others.

6. Perform the solar meditation cleaning for the next 5 minutes or until you feel completely cleaned.

A Heart Chakra Meditation Method

1. You will begin by finding a location or ground that is peaceful and comfortable, with no potential for disruptions. Sit with your back straight, breathe with your nose, and exhale through your mouth. Inhale and exhale for at least 5 to 10 minutes or more, relaxing your body while you do so. Imagine bringing green energy up through your body to your heart, starting at the bottom of your body and working your

way up to your heart and out. See that green energy brightening and expanding as you inhale and exhale, and imagine it as a dazzling, gigantic green ball.

2. Focus on offering yourself and others love and compassion while allowing the green energy to flow through your body and repeat these meditation techniques for at least 5 minutes or longer.

3. Cleansing and focusing on the present moment

4. This type of cleansing is essential, especially if you want to eliminate the countless difficulties in your life.

5. Close your eyes and take a long breath in before exhaling slowly.

6. Consider everything in your life, including your negative thoughts, what others think of you, and your ideas about who you are or who you want to be, and set them aside.

7. Take all of your past and look at the present, the chances accessible to you, and what you want to achieve and execute.

8. If you notice any tension in your thoughts, such as what you desire to happen, or if they are unreasonable, let them go.

Now that your perspective is clear, be open to new ideas and enable yourself to be filled with good and clear thinking.

Meditation with Unifying Phrases

The brain is responsible for most human suffering. Meditation helps us relax and be open to ourselves to rid ourselves of negative or stressful ideas and fill ourselves with pleasant energy and thoughts. Unifying meditation is an affirmation that covers a suffering mind and ideas. The unifying phrase allows you to entirely shift your focus away from unpleasant and negative ideas and energy in your being to open the door to positive and gratifying thoughts.

By shifting your ideas and mentality, you will be able to quickly get rid of negative thoughts and memories and replace them with good and positive energy and recollections.

1. Begin by shutting your eyes or leaving them open, inhaling deeply, and exhaling smoothly while repeating the unifying words below.

2. "I allow myself to accept everything as it is right now."

3. "I am attentive and aware of everything going on around me."

4. "I like tranquility."

5. "I'm at peace with my maker."

The unifying meditation can also be spiritual, to choose to side with your creator and all that is good and positive.

Ways to Boost Your Healing Process

We all require clear energy to flow through us. Without that healthy energy running through your chakras, you will feel unhappy and empty, as if someone had cut the power to everything you have ever desired. If you have a blockage in your energy centers, it will seem like a power outage, but you can take action to clear them. You will never lose your strength. All you have to do is re-establish the flow.

You embody a complicated system from your root chakra at your tailbone to your crown chakra at the top of your head. In a healthy cycle, this system gets energy from the surrounding environment and returns energy to it. When your energy centers are balanced and free of obstructions, they spin miniature wheels that keep you healthy. Blockages to the free movement of your chakras can occur over time due to emotional disturbances, daily living, and trauma.

You will discover several methods for healing your chakras. However, to ensure that those strategies function to their full potential, the following seven actions might assist in supercharging your energy cleansing activities. They are all really simple and can be completed by anyone.

Return to Earth

Spend some time outside with nature. Go for a lengthy stroll in the park or go hiking. If you can remove your shoes and walk barefoot for a bit, you will lay a new foundation for yourself. It will assist you in grounding into your surroundings and reconnecting with the earth. Time spent outside will leave you feeling present, protected and will assist in developing your root chakra.

Immerse Yourself in Healing Waters

This is perfect if you can get to the beach and immerse yourself in the water. Fill a bathtub halfway with water, sea salt, and baking soda if you can't. This will aid in the strengthening of your sacral chakra. Your sexual chakra is in charge of your joys, and feelings of shame and guilt readily taint it. Imagine all of your feelings of shame and guilt vanishing while you swim as the water strives to restore the purity of your actual nature.

Move

When you move your body, your solar plexus chakra rejoices. It enjoys being outside in the sunlight of a newly rising sun or just as the sun sets. Any physical exercise can enable you to awaken and cleanse your third chakra, which will give you greater willpower, self-esteem, and personal strength.

Accept and Share Love

Your heart chakra is the key to your compassion, and it rejoices when you receive unconditional love. This love may be love for yourself, love for others, love for everyone, and love for the globe. Spend some time with your pet in a way that demonstrates reciprocal affection. This is an excellent technique to ensure that you receive a healthy dosage of compassion in your life. Even if you don't have a pet, it's not difficult to find methods to feel compassion and love. You may volunteer at your local animal shelter.

Make Your Voice Heard

When you don't allow yourself to express yourself, your throat chakra suffers. The fifth chakra empowers you to speak up and be yourself. If you don't want to say something, write it down in a notebook and be honest about it. Nobody else is going to read it, so express yourself freely. It will not only relieve tension but will also activate your throat chakra. Turn on some music and sing your heart out when you have some spare time alone (or not alone if your buddies don't mind). This will also aid in opening up your fifth chakra. Communicate honestly while speaking with someone.

Pay Attention to Your Inner Self

Your higher self resides in your Third Eye and supplies you with clarity. Daily meditation practice is critical to repairing your energy and chakras. It will also activate your sixth chakra, allowing you to transform into the wisdom you already possess. You will notice that you begin to place greater confidence in your intuition. Meditation will assist you in removing the mental noise that you must deal with daily, allowing you to view things more clearly.

Contact with the Spirit

Your crown chakra connects you to the cosmos and your higher abilities. It is in charge of your awareness. Meditation, which strengthens the Third Eye chakra, is an excellent approach to connect with higher powers and stimulate the seventh chakra. Prayer is another approach to clean up your top chakra. This prayer may be whatever you want it to be. You can pray to the universe, God, or anybody you want. It might simply be a simple slogan that you repeat every day. Taking time to connect with nature may also aid in the cleansing and charging your head chakra or any of your chakras. Every day, communicate with your higher power and ask for direction. Visualize calm and happy results for whatever is going on in your life or the globe.

As you focus on balancing and cleansing your chakras, you will feel better and have more energy flowing through you. Your chakra system will take in and release energy as it should. When everything is in sync, you will feel healthier and happier.

The Risks of Chakra Activation

We've talked about your chakras and what they do for your body. We've also discussed the symptoms of chakra blockage and the advantages of opening them. Before you begin working on your chakras, you should be aware of the hazards of over-opening them.

There are several reasons to direct your energy toward your chakras and ensure they are open and functioning properly. When your heart chakra is balanced, it will aid you in all of your relationships. When your throat chakra is open, you may speak your truth. Making your chakras a priority is wonderful but moving too quickly might have negative implications.

More energy will enter you when your chakras are open. Blocked chakras generate stuck energy that will not flow easily through you. Blockages must be eliminated, but this must be done gradually. Going too rapidly will result in a lot of energy being absorbed.

What occurs when you open your chakras too rapidly depends on which chakra you are opening and how much energy you are utilizing. Consider what the chakra performs for you to find this out.

As you are aware, the heart chakra governs your ability to love. You may avoid partnerships if your heart chakra is obstructed. When you open your heart chakra too rapidly, a surge of energy may overwhelm you and send your heart chakra into overdrive. This might make you clingy in your relationships. You may also find yourself bonding with individuals too easily. As a result, the chakra is no better than before it was blocked.

When your Third Eye chakra is blocked, you lose contact with your intuition. You rely on intellect and do not listen to your intuition. If you open this one too quickly, you will be flooded with energy, which will overwhelm you and the chakra. You may end up having frightening intuitions. You could develop psychic talents that you can't control. Spirits from other realms may begin to communicate with you, and you will be unable to control them. Again, this leaves your chakra in the same condition when blocked.

While this may appear frightening, it does not imply you should avoid opening them altogether. Instead, all you need to do is open them slowly. When it comes to chakra opening, you want to be the turtle, not the hare.

You should avoid anything or anybody who promises to help you fast awaken your chakras. You must be patient. You must have faith that your chakras will open on their own time, without you having to go to extremes.

When you open your chakras, you may experience many distinct side effects. The majority will only occur if you allow them to open too soon.

Detachment

When your crown chakra is open, this might happen. When you go on a spiritual trip to work with your chakras or any spiritual journey, you are usually relatively alone. Each of us must travel our path. Many people will notice that they prefer to be alone, especially if the head chakra opens too soon. This may leave you feeling detached.

Déjà Vu

This might occur with your crown chakra and Third Eye chakra. While this is generally an indication that a chakra has been effectively opened, it can also occur in excess, indicating that you opened them too rapidly. This may be overpowering, and it can also flow over into your dreams, resulting in vivid or terrifying dreams.

Disruptions in Sleep

After healing their chakras, many people notice that they don't sleep as much. This also implies that if you open them too rapidly, it may create sleep disturbances. You could discover that you can't feel comfy when sleeping. All of this might lead to feelings of irritability and instability.

Overstimulated Senses

This is frequently the result of an overworked root chakra. When the root chakra opens, you become more aware of the ground, including how it feels, sounds, looks, and smells. You will be inundated with these sensations if you open that chakra too rapidly. You could even find it difficult to function because the sun is too bright, or you smell the flowery scent of the lady five seats behind you on the bus. It may drive you insane with everything you start sensing.

Bladder Abnormalities and Reproductive Difficulties

This is common when the sacral chakra is hyperactive. This might result in lower abdominal aches and pains, atypical bladder habits, and urine issues. It may also have an impact on women's menstrual cycles. If not treated, it can lead to more significant endometriosis, testicular or prostate problems, ovarian cysts, and infertility.

Anger Issues

When your solar plexus chakra is hyperactive, you may experience more rage than normal. This might imply that you are upset for no apparent cause or go off the handle at the drop of a hat. This might also include developing a new sense of perfectionism and being too critical of yourself and others.

Emotional Neglect

If you allow your chakras to expand too soon, you may become too focused on caring for others. This will lead to you neglecting yourself, which will lead to even more difficulties.

Meditation is an excellent approach to help repair your chakras gradually so that you do not become overwhelmed. Another technique to set an intention to restore your chakras is via prayer. Wearing gems that help you balance your chakras is a fantastic idea. These gems will gradually boost your vibration and alter the energy surrounding your chakras. Color therapy is another excellent method for balancing your chakras.

Healing anything takes time, and this is especially true for chakra healing. Allowing things to happen on their own will allow you to see a change that will not leave you feeling overwhelmed.

Mistakes People Make

You will see tremendous results if you know how to correctly use your chakras and energy. People frequently make the following seven blunders when attempting to restore their chakras.

As the earth undergoes a spiritual awakening, more individuals turn to energy healing activities. Occasionally, though, things do not proceed as intended, or something interferes. Energy healing is meant to bring about observable improvements in your life. This may include anything from your real emotions to your belief systems.

Most of the time, the changes that occur due to this type of treatment are said to be miraculous, but this only occurs if everything goes as planned. If your healing isn't miraculous, you could be making one of these blunders.

You Should Stop When You Feel Better

Energy or chakra healing is similar to medications in that you must continue even after you start feeling better. You must continue to heal when you are happy and sad. You won't get the whole experience if you don't.

You must be able to deal with problems even when you feel better. Dive into your concerns and reach the layers that will create the most significant adjustments. This implies your system will be able to manage additional workload.

Working on your chakras daily, especially while you are in a good mood, may help you anticipate and prevent terrible circumstances. This will help you live a more peaceful existence, which you were aiming for in the first place.

Failure to Maintain

Like any other system, your chakras require regular maintenance, or they will become blocked again. If you only work on things while in a crisis, your body will focus on the subject at hand and ignore everything else. You will be able to maintain your chakras clean and in alignment with each other if you have frequent sessions, preventing energy back up.

Attempting to Heal Bodily Issues

Chakra healing benefits you on many levels: spiritually, psychologically, physically, and emotionally. However, many individuals cleanse their chakras just to alleviate physical discomfort. This is merely a subset of what chakra healing can achieve, so there's no use in limiting oneself to only addressing physical issues. Increase the number of reasons you have for doing things in your life.

Inadequate Time Management

After working with your chakras, you may see a few quick outcomes in various areas. You should expect things to move and change in three weeks when you first start. This means you won't see outcomes as quickly as you had anticipated. This can make you believe nothing is working and convince you to give up.

To fix this, keep a daily journal where you write down how you are feeling.

Waiting Until Issues Have Passed

This might happen straight away as you begin to repair your chakras, or it could happen a few weeks later, but you will be unwell or have a lot of symptoms. Don't let this stop you from continuing to recover. These are the times when you need it. Healing sessions can assist you in pushing past these difficulties and achieving new levels of vitality.

Whether you're unwell or a lot is going on, most problems are caused by your energy change. The bad energy must be moved elsewhere to be released. You'll be surprised at how great you'll feel if you keep working through these issues while healing.

Constantly Whining

Humans have a penchant for whining. It's also too simple for us to become engrossed in a concept and pick at it, breaking it down and analyzing it repeatedly. After doing some healing work, you will go through a 24- to 72-hour phase in which your old energy will migrate out of your body. This might emerge in a variety of ways.

If you think about something you're worried about all the time, it will just reinforce the problem and those pathways, trapping it in your system. This prevents it from being removed from your system after a therapeutic session.

Not Believing

Astonishment and disbelief are common reactions to hearing about or experiencing chakra healing's ability. Because your mind creates your reality, it will build your world in everything.

If you don't believe that chakra healing works, it won't work for you. Energy healing works in conjunction with your belief system. That is why you must ensure that your belief system and therapeutic work are in sync. When you tell yourself repeatedly that you don't believe it will work, you will simply unravel your efforts.

If you can avoid these typical blunders, you will get the advantages of chakra healing.

CHAPTER 19: THE THIRD EYE & OPENING IT

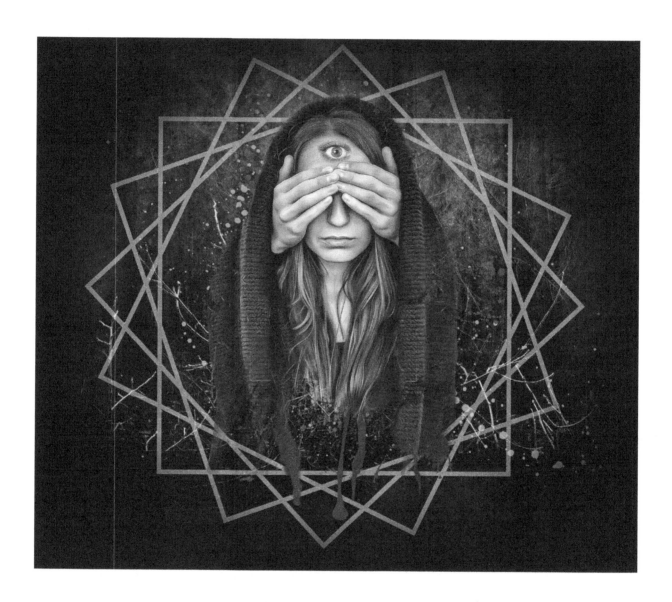

What is the Third Eye?

The "Third Eye" refers to both a physical and spiritual portion of the body. In its physical appearance, the pineal gland is a gland located at the top of the spine that links to the brain. Physiologically, this endocrine gland serves a variety of functions within the body. Outside of scientific circles, it is commonly referred to as the Third Eye. If you were to regard someone in the face straight, the pineal gland would be directly above both eyes, right in the middle, like another eye, therefore its name.

The pineal gland secretes hormones such as melatonin and serotonin, which are important in regulating sleep patterns and contributing to the general mood. Without this gland, the body would be unable to detect typical oscillations in light, making it difficult to fall and stay asleep in a normal pattern. Aside from the temperature difference, the body would be unable to distinguish between summer and winter. The pineal gland is found in the majority of vertebrate species and so keeps the entire ecosystem operating on the same clock, which is dependent on sunlight.

Activating and Sustaining Third-Eye Function

In Hindu and Ayurvedic beliefs, specific mudras, or mantras, are claimed to assist, activate and sustain the health of each chakra. Chanting "OM" in a peaceful environment for 1–20 minutes is advised for the Third Eye chakra. Musical compositions are intended to resonate with each chakra based on its unique tonal frequency. The Third Eye chakra's frequencies are 144 Hz, 288 Hz, and 576 Hz.

Meditation is by far the most popular method for opening the Third Eye. While there are many different types of meditation, the general aim is to slow down the cognitive process. How often have we had the term for something on the tip of our tongue, but the more we attempt to remember it, the more difficult it is to recall? And then, after we've gotten our minds off it, the word comes to us effortlessly and instantaneously!

Because many effective meditation practitioners have stated its objective as bringing cognitive awareness to higher levels of brain function where theta and delta waves are separate, sleep phases and brain waves are included. It is believed that we learn control over stress reduction and our bodies' healing processes as observed naturally occurring in Stage IV sleep.

Dr. Nipun Aggarwal, MD, MBA, MHT, and José Silva are two well-known authorities who have developed ways to "mind control," which involve teaching our mind's eye to deliberately, effectively, and almost quickly manage body activities for optimal health. These tactics are also targeted at retaining focus and peace of mind in demanding and hard everyday situations, memorizing and swiftly retrieving huge quantities of information, and fluent problem solving beyond our five senses.

Using the Third Eye does not imply that you will gain magical abilities or become a psychic. It means being able to govern your thoughts more efficiently and having a stronger sense of intuition about your surroundings. Unfortunately, this transition does not happen overnight; you will need to devote your life to spiritual activities that include the daily practice of mind awareness.

The First Opening

Choose a day when you will have a lot of free time, such as the start of a weekend. This allows you to concentrate on the eye-opening techniques in more depth. After the initial opening, it usually becomes simpler. You may do it with buddies or by yourself. It is best to dress in bright colors. The first opening isn't particularly strong; you could feel a tingle between your brows.

Technique

1. Go to a quiet, peaceful location where you won't be interrupted for at least an hour.
2. Place candles all around the place.
3. Take off your shoes, watch, tie, belt, and other constricting apparel or jewelry.
4. Lie down on the floor, carpet, blanket, or mat with your arms at your sides and palms up.
5. Close your eyes for 3 minutes, relax for 3 minutes, and then hum for 5 to 10 minutes.

Phase 1

- Begin breathing via the throat, becoming aware of the vibration within the larynx as you do.
- Continue to breathe for 5 to 10 minutes, and if your body or consciousness moves, allow it to.

Phase 2

- While sustaining the throat friction, direct your attention to the area between your brows.
- You must flow with the energy of your body. Pay no attention to the time.

Phase 3

- Place your palm about 3 to 5 cm away from the region between the brows.

Phase 4

- You might have your hand in phase 3 or by your side.
- Begin to seek vibration or tingle between the brows with your eyes closed and your larynx vibrating.
- You may also notice a hazy pressure, density, or weight.
- Don't try to concentrate too hard; instead, stay void and let things take their natural course.

Phase 5

- When you sense vibration or anything between your brows, attempt to associate it with the friction in your neck.
- The vibration will progressively get more subtle while also becoming stronger.
- Some people may experience vibrations in other portions of their bodies or throughout their forehead. This is normal; just concentrate on the vibration between your brows.

Phase 6

- Put a stop to the vibration in the larynx.
- Pay attention to the vibration between the brows.
- Stay quiet, motionless, and attempt to concentrate on the energy surrounding you.
- Keep an eye out for any light or colors between the brows.

Remember

- Throughout the procedure, keep your eyes closed.
- Do not grab or focus too much on the area between the brows since this may obstruct the process.
- Do not touch each other if you are training with pals.
- If the experience becomes too much for you, open your eyes to return to normal awareness.

The expressions of the eye are not as critical for the first encounter as getting the method properly. Little physical movements such as twitching and flashing in and out of awareness are possible during the first opening. Ignore them and continue to develop your technique as if nothing had happened.

How to Learn to Meditate

To begin, you must locate the appropriate environment. Choose a location that allows you to be alone for at least 30 to 45 minutes and is quite calm. It doesn't have to be silent but try to locate a location where you won't be disturbed too much.

Assume a Meditative Posture

A particularly efficient position is sitting on the ground with crossed legs, straight back, and hands resting on the knees. If you can't sit on the ground, sit on a chair with your back straight. Use your abdominal muscles to support your upper body and avoid slouching your back. Maintain a relaxed posture with your shoulders down and your chest out.

Relax Your Body

We all carry stress in our bodies while going about our everyday lives, making it difficult to focus. You won't notice how stiff your muscles are unless you try to relax them intentionally. Roll your head from side to side to relax your muscles and allow your shoulders to drop.

Unwind Your Mind

This is one of the most important steps towards opening the Third Eye. It may also be the most difficult since you need to clear your mind of all ideas. You may accomplish this by concentrating your attention on any one component of the physical environment, such as the sensation of the earth beneath your feet, the sound of passing traffic, or the in and out of your breath.

While it is difficult to eradicate all ideas, simply notice them and let them pass if one does enter your mind. To clear your mind, you will need a lot of patience and practice. People find it challenging to meditate during the first 10 to 20 minutes. Allow yourself some time to move from the outside world to a contemplative state.

Create a Habit of Meditating

The more you think about it, the better you'll get at it. You may think about meditation while eating, walking, or brushing your teeth. Even if you only meditate for 5 minutes every day, you will train yourself to become more attentive and thoughtful over time. While meditating, set a timer to avoid worrying about how much time you've already spent meditating.

Activate Your Brain's Intuitive Part

Begin by taking in your surroundings. People who are normally shy are more intuitive than the average person because they spend a lot of time studying other people. As a result, they better know things like facial expression, body language, and other forms of non-explicit communication. These individuals are adept at sensing sexual chemistry, deception, hidden signals, and sarcasm.

You may exercise intuition by traveling to a public location on your own, such as a café, restaurant, or park, and simply observing the people around you. Try not to be overpowering or disrespectful when listening in on their chat. Imagine a tale about how these individuals met, what they're talking about, or any other information that piques your curiosity. The more you practice, the better you'll get.

You may also practice it when sitting around the table with your friends or family; try remaining silent and simply listening to what they are saying. People who are not engaging in the conversation should be observed, and their reactions to the continuing dialogue should be observed. Consider what they could be thinking while they are not speaking. The more you practice, the better you will get.

Dreams are Essential

According to people with psychic abilities, dreams can include messages that might act as a warning. Begin by writing down your dreams to evaluate them. The easiest method to accomplish this is to keep a dream journal next to your pillow after documenting a few dreams, attempting to establish links between them, and seeing whether they have come true.

Follow Your Gut Instincts

Have you ever had a strange feeling about a location, event, or person that you couldn't quite put into words? Have you ever felt that a specific circumstance may occur, but you didn't have any proof to back it up? These sensations are known as gut instincts, and we all experience them to varying degrees. Most individuals disregard their gut impulses and attempt to conduct their life based on logic. Make a note of it the next time you experience such a feeling and see if it comes true. Also, consider whether these sentiments have any relevance to your life.

Remember that just because you have a gut feeling about something doesn't imply it will come true. While it may come true, it may take months or even years for it to occur, which is why it is always beneficial to keep a record of these sensations so that when it does, you know for certain that you were aware of it.

Experiences Following the Third Eye's Opening

You will have some unexpected experiences once your Third Eye opens. While many of the events will be enjoyable, others may not be. If you sense activity or pressure in the center of your forehead, this indicates that your Third Eye has already opened or will open shortly.

Seeing with the Third Eye

The Third Eye allows you to look beyond the visual pictures surrounding you. You may use it to detect and visually understand the energy around you. You will learn much more than just the abstract notion of random individuals strolling in the park if you observe people walking in the park. In a vivid internal visual map, you see the interplay between motion, energy, and purpose. As a result, life becomes palpable to you.

While our physical eyes are blind to energy and can only observe its effects, the Third Eye allows us to envision where the energy is, comprehend it, and see it. Our eyes are intended to sense light. However, the Third Eye assists you in processing the energy with which you engage in a precise manner.

Having an open Third Eye may appear magical at first, but it is simply a new way for your mind to interact with the rest of your senses. This communication is so direct and unrestrained that it allows you to precisely forecast occurrences and detect potentials that are not physically there. This is a genuine technique that has been practiced by humanity since the Paleolithic epoch.

What to Expect When the Third Eye Opens

Do not be astonished if you have any unexpected encounters once your Third Eye has opened. This will have a big impact on what you see. For example, if you are weary after a hard day's work and are going to sleep, you may see many sights in your mind's eye after closing your actual eyes.

Many of these visuals will be blurry or vibrant and make little sense. With an open Third Eye, you may gradually go to various dimensions you will discover. It all relies on the vibration levels of your thoughts. The more dimensions you can explore, the higher your vibration levels. If you see blurry visions, you'll need to boost your spiritual powers. A greater level of meditation will allow you to see more clearly with your Third Eye.

Dimensions: Upper and Lower

If your thoughts have low vibrations, you will witness images from a lower realm. The lowest dimension is where you'll find restless spirits. These are the souls of persons who either murdered themselves or couldn't forgive themselves for anything they did in their lifetimes. They do not enter the upper plane because they are terrified of being judged.

People who encounter sights from the bottom realm are usually terrified of what they see and regret activating their Third Eye. However, you are not required to stay in the lower dimension. Most people who stay in the lower dimension do so because the vibration generated by their thoughts pulls them there. You have to raise your frequency and enter a higher dimension.

If you want to close your Third Eye, shun spiritual activities, engage in discussions that have nothing to do with the spiritual realm, and get rid of everything in your environment that reminds you of it. While your Third Eye may not close immediately, it will do so gradually. However, it is crucial to remember that it will require a lot of work to open it again once your Third Eye closes.

Higher thought vibrations, such as sentiments of pleasure, appreciation, love, or peace, can allow you to view more tranquil visions, bringing your spirit a sense of fulfillment and comfort. In this realm, you will receive images of the pain that others are experiencing, solutions to assist you in making circumstances better, and sentiments of compassion and forgiveness.

Sensitivity to Positive and Negative Energies

When your Third Eye is activated, you will become more sensitive to the energy of others around you. You will be able to tell the difference between good and harmful energy. It's always a good idea to take up positive vibes since they will benefit you. However, it is hard to prevent picking up terrible energy, so it is always good to avoid situations where you know harmful energies may impact you. This is one of the primary reasons people with higher spiritual abilities feel fatigued after spending time in a crowd since they are bombarded with negative energy.

To defend yourself when you're amid negative energy. Think of anything that makes you joyful and keep doing it until you can get out of that situation. It will prevent your mind from being entangled in unpleasant ideas.

Once you've gotten out of that circumstance and returned home, take a shower at a slightly lower temperature than you're used to. Imagine the water washing away all of the negative energy that has afflicted you. Feel the negative energy go down with the water as it flows from your body. This is an excellent exercise for removing the effects of negative energy from your mind. You will notice a stronger cleaning impact after a few days of using it. It will also help you become more focused and energetic throughout the day, and negative energies will lose their ability to disrupt your regular thought process. It will also enhance your quality of life, health, sleep, relationships, and overall mental condition.

Third Eye Opening Observations

After your Third Eye has opened, you may experience high-level vibrations that are frightening at first. The key to getting through this moment is to remain quiet and let the vibrations take control of your thoughts. Remain calm, and your mind will coordinate with the vibrations and get accustomed to them.

You may have visions of beautiful places, such as a beautiful day or a beautiful house, or anything else that you believe is a very peaceful and enlightening place to be. Even if you are not physically there in such a location, your mind will reap all of the benefits of being there. The magnitude of the visuals you see in your vision will vary depending on your level of focus and meditation. While certain visions may be in a frame, causing the mind to be aware of the darkness surrounding the frame, others may be frameless, with such clarity that the mind no longer sees any darkness or problematic pictures.

Third Eye Closure

Many people may decide to close their Third Eye. For some, the sensations that follow waking and activation of it can be overpowering. The simplest method to keep it closed in such circumstances is to avoid using it. Opening the eye necessitates effort and modifications in your daily routine. When you conduct commonplace and pointless actions that don't necessitate the employment of the Third Eye, it closes on its own. Just maintain your attention on the steady flow of events.

Simply push yourself back and become more anchored in the present for individuals who have opened their Third Eye. Continue to direct your attention to where you are and what is around you. You can regulate what you see and hear, even if you start seeing and hearing more. Simply prevent yourself from seeing or hearing what you don't want to see or hear. It's as simple as closing your eyes or changing the station on the television when you don't want to see anything. Increase your awareness of your physical presence and style of living. This will keep you grounded and prevent you from experiencing greater realms of consciousness. Don't let your mind wander to things that are too profound and have little to do with your daily existence. All of this contributes to a reduction in Third Eye awareness.

CHAPTER 20: YOUR DIVINE BEING

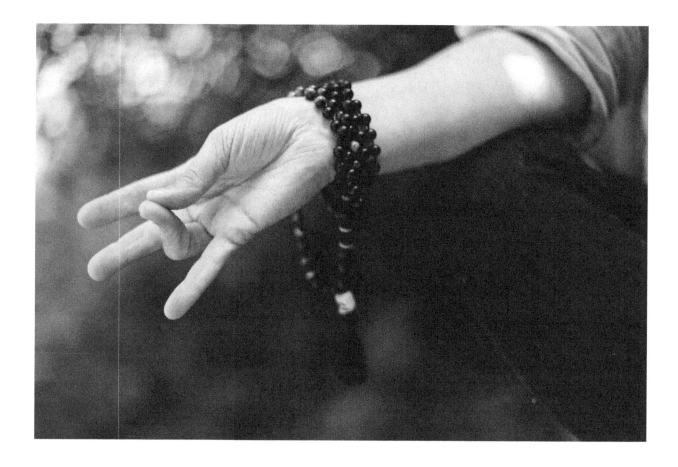

The inner life energy is the divine self. This is your genuine reason for being alive. You are awestruck by the divine self's might. The light in your center decided to be incarnate at a specific point in time.

The divine self is constantly conscious. It has been thinking and conscious since you were born in this and every previous existence. The physical environment and body we live in are only containers for your higher self.

You choose to be here, which is why you are. This dynamic force of consciousness and life gives you lessons to learn and exchanges to make that you are only about to do as a person.

It may appear that the norms of incarnation, birth, and life in this hectic world would keep us from recognizing our divine self, which is within our core. This does not have to be the case. You have the option to change it.

We may recognize our divine essence and begin to pull ourselves closer to our higher being.

The first thing you must do is accept your divine nature. Allow your thoughts to shut down as you quiet and relax.

Remove any distractions. There should be no music, clocks, phones, children, lawnmowers, television, or radios.

Choose a mirror or a candle to sit in front of. Look into the flame if you choose a candle. If you choose to utilize a mirror, begin by looking over your complete face. Don't gaze into your eyes, and don't let the flame cause your eyes to go out of focus.

Maintain self-awareness. Stay in your body and remain comfortable. Maintain your attention. The candle flame depicts the light that is the source of all life. Light powers everything that is living. The absorption and reflection of light make all things perceptible. All that exists is light. The mirror portrays a self-image that is both shunned and welcomed. We avoid it because we want to compare it to the beauty or perfection we anticipate finding in the natural world. We avoid flaws in our appearance because they make us feel unlovable and inadequate.

People fail to see that life is all about flaws. Conscious energy is flawless and longs to be incarnated so that it might experience the sadness and joy of life. It wants to feel imperfect sadness and joy and learn how to offer unconditional love in the face of these tragedies and imperfections.

This is the one period in your life when you may acquire meaningful lessons and go closer to merging with the All. The Source or Creator is the All. It is neither feminine nor masculine but just is. Everything is presented in the same manner as everything else; it is derived from its source. This indicates that everyone, consciousness, and light are always present, and everyone is a part of the Light Family.

We often overlook that the objects and people we believe are flawless have been altered to appear perfect, and they are not natural. Natural perfection is a figment of one's imagination.

Another reason we embrace ourselves is the ego; everyone realizes that we have a body with a form, face, mouth, nose, and eyes. We believe this because we are about to witness and feel it for ourselves.

When a person looks in a mirror, they are likely to simply perceive a physical item, something composed of matter, like a candle or a match. We are matter that deteriorate and die, yet there is more to us. We may be angry, love, weep, create things with our hands, celebrate faiths, reproduce, stay up late thinking, and make decisions.

Is it enough that we exist? Are we not more akin to a personality embodied or a spirit?

Thoughts and personalities are more than simply bodily functions. A bodily function may power them, but this is just a link between your body and soul. An automobile is powered by gas through combustion, which alters the condition of the gas. The intellect attempts to convert the spirit, but we require the spirit to live. When our motor clogs, we merely need to check for a neglected spirit to figure out why.

Consider your reflection in the mirror to be more than simply bone and flesh, but also a spiritual being that moves within your body. Then you will deepen your connection to things beyond the physical realm.

Take a peek at yourself in the mirror. Take note of your body's brightness and the life-giving glow surrounding it.

Embrace the energy of creation, the light of life, and your connection to it while doing this with the mirror or candle. Say to yourself, "I believe in myself. I know because I feel it in my body. I've seen it in my own life."

Repeat after me, and don't be a slacker. Repeat as many times as you sense this truth in your heart. Take notice of the divine energy and connection to the cosmos and the buzz of creation on your skin.

Continue to do so or adjust it to suit your needs. Consider the divine self, and then make contact with the manifesting self.

Keep your heart open to the divine self and your divine self to be able to speak with the higher being and watch how your life unfolds.

Do the same with the moon's cycle. This is most effective during a new moon. Continue doing this for as long as you feel you need to strengthen your relationship with your higher being and better know it.

The higher self lies at the mystical center of all faiths. Understanding one's higher self is the most valuable asset someone can have.

On the Chart of Your Divine Self, the higher self is portrayed as having a relationship with the evolving self. I demonstrate numerous cosmic truths uncovered by great mystics of the West and East.

The chart is divided into three sections, referred to as your identity's trinity.

A sphere of light is housed in an upper figure. This is referred to as Brahma by Hindus. Buddhists refer to it as Dharmakaya, while Christians refer to it as the Heavenly Father. God's spirit has been customized for each person.

Your higher self is encompassed by the seven spheres of your physical body. All of your positive works are contained within these energy spheres. This is your heavenly bank account.

Your body has seven planes of heaven and seven fields of awareness, which correlate to the seven days of creation, the seven archangels, the seven Elohim, and the seven hues that emanate from the white light that is the Father.

These seven routes lead to seven paths that return to the Source. The seven ray lords are masters who teach on these pathways.

Your higher self is already a part of you. It will never be taken down. It does not exist in space or time apart from you. The only thing standing between you and your higher self is your consciousness, limits, and the vibrations you've gathered from this and prior lives that are less than your highest attributes.

The higher self exists between the light above and the soul below. The higher self is a part of you that transforms a flawed soul into a flawless one. It is a genuine part of you that can stand in the face of your God.

Some Christians refer to your higher self as the man's inner heart. Your higher self is the one who guides you through your evolutions and all of your encounters in space and time.

Depending on your faith, you can think of your higher self as a guardian angel, conscience, inner guru, and best friend.

The chart demonstrates that we all have a higher self and are destined to be one with that higher self. It makes no difference whether we call it Atman, Tao, Buddha, or Christ.

In space and time, your soul progresses on a spiritual journey. It is a component of your mortal self, yet it has the potential to become eternal.

The violet flame is a presence that envelops you. This flame is high-frequency energy that forgives. It is a type of spiritual alchemy.

Around the violet flame is a protecting white light known as God. We use the spoken word to summon the light for safety. It will protect our chakras and aura from the heaviness of the darkness.

The silver or umbilical cord is the white light that descends from God to the higher self. It's your rope to the Spirit. This silver wire nurtures a dazzling light of God that is sealed inside the heart's secret chamber. This is a three-fold flame with love, knowledge, and power qualities. It is a very spiritual flame about 1/16th of an inch in diameter and is centered in the body's heart. God has transferred a sacred fire from his heart to yours.

The goal of your incarnations is to become your true self to return to the spiritual plane, which is your true home. Your soul's goal is to rise to the light, complete your purpose, balance your karma, and gain self-mastery. Paying attention to your spiritual journey will finally unite the figures on the chart that are split owing to a restricted consciousness.

CHAPTER 21: MINDFUL MEDITATION & GETTING RID OF NEGATIVE ENERGY

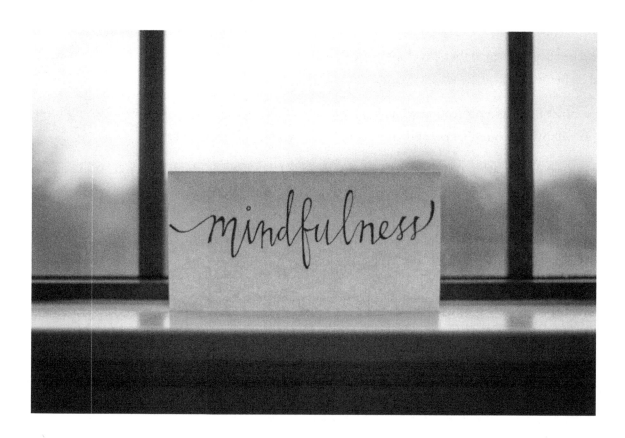

Mindful Meditation

Mindful meditation is an essential sort of meditation. Mindfulness is the discipline of paying attention to what is going on in the present moment, which you may learn by practice and meditation.

In Buddhist teachings, mindfulness leads to spiritual enlightenment and the end of suffering.

Lots of research on mindfulness have been conducted, and they have discovered that it may help you live a better, happier life. When you spend your life worrying and obsessing about things you can't control or that will happen in the future, you're living in the negative, leading to anxiety, depression, and other mental diseases.

Begin by practicing mindfulness meditation for 10 minutes every day for the first several sessions. Once you've gotten the hang of it, try increasing the duration by five- or ten-minutes increments, whatever you believe you'll be able to accomplish effectively. The objective is to get to 30 minutes of exercise every day. You can rehearse for a longer period, but it is not required.

Mindfulness aims to educate you on how to live in the present moment. While you may believe you already do, consider where your mind is when you're living. Do you taste your food and appreciate what it does for your body when eating breakfast? Most likely not. Mindfulness teaches you how to have your mind and body working in tandem.

The Buddhist tradition is the finest location to learn about mindfulness. The term mindfulness is derived from the Pali word *sati* and the Sanskrit word *smriti*. Smriti means "to remember," or "to recall." Sati also means "to recall."

Now that you know what mindfulness is, let's look at some meditations to get you started living thoughtfully.

3 Minutes – Body and Sound

Begin by paying attention to your current posture. You might be seated, standing, or lying down. Take note of how your body feels right now. Now try to observe the feelings present in your body at this time.

You may have a sense of lightness or heaviness, weight, or pressure. You could even feel chilly, heated, move, pulsate, or vibrate. These feelings might be felt everywhere in your body. All you have to do is pay attention to them.

Take note of these details with interest and inquiry. Take a long, deep breath in. Allow your body to relax as you breathe in. Do nothing but remain present and aware of your body.

Allow all of those sensations to subside. Now pay attention to the sounds around you. These can be located either inside or outside of your room. There might be a wide range of noises. Sounds might be quiet or loud. You should also pay attention to the quiet that occurs between the noises. Take note of how the sound fades in and out.

The mind has a propensity to focus on certain noises. It begins to create a tale for the sound. Or you believe you must respond to it: I don't like that, I like that.

Rather, see if you can just listen. Take note of it with wonder and attention. The noises are coming and departing.

Return your attention to your body, which is currently standing, laying, or seated. Take note of any noticeable physical feelings. Take a deep breath again. Allow your body to relax. When you're ready, gradually open your eyes.

9 Minutes – Loving Meditation

Allow yourself to feel calm and at ease where you are seated before beginning this meditation. You will create pleasant feelings, notably loving compassion, with this exercise. You want someone to be happy, or you want to be happy.

This is neither conditional nor dependent on anything. This is simply letting your heart open to yourself or another person. Take this opportunity to check in with yourself and observe how you feel. Allow whatever is present to be present.

Allow your thoughts to come up with something. This should include someone who makes you joyful just thinking about them. See if you can think of anyone. This might be a friend or a family member. It's preferable if it's someone with whom you have a simple relationship. It should just be a basic feeling you get when they come to mind. You may even select a child.

You can select a pet instead of a human if you have difficulty thinking of someone. Any animal that is simple to fall in love with. Allow them to enter your thoughts.

It's as though they're standing right in front of you. They can be seen, felt, and sensed. Take notice of how you feel on the inside while you visualize this. You could feel the heat, or your face might feel heated. You might also begin to smile or feel more spacious. This is an act of loving compassion.

This sensation is normal, and everyone can experience it at any time. Begin wishing your loved one well now that you have them in front of you. I wish them safety and protection from harm. I wish them peace and happiness. I wish them strength and health. I wish them happiness and comfort. You may either wish them precisely what I said or use your own words.

Take note of how you allow this loving-kindness to emanate from you and how your loved one impacts you.

You may see images in your head, notice light or color, or experience a mood during this time. More of these sentiments might be triggered by your words to a loved one. Say whatever is most important to you. I wish for them to be free of tension, anxiety, and fear.

Check in with yourself to observe how you feel when you offer them these words and sentiments of loving compassion. Imagine your loved one has turned around and has begun to convey these emotions back to you. See if you can receive and absorb their wonderful goodness.

They want you to be happy. Therefore, they wish you well. This includes you. I wish you happiness and tranquility. I wish you protection and safety from every harm. I wish you happiness and health.

Allow yourself to absorb this. It's not a huge issue if you haven't started to experience this loving-kindness yet or never felt it in past meditations. This procedure entails planting seeds. Check in with yourself if you start to feel something other than loving compassion. What exactly are you feeling? This emotion may teach you anything.

If you're ready, and it won't always be easy, try sending yourself some love. This might be visualized as a light streaming down your body from your heart. All you need is a feeling for it. Say to yourself, "I want to be secure and protected. I want to be healthy and robust. I want to be at peace and joyful. I want to accept myself as I am."

Then ask yourself, "What will make me happy?" Take note of what arises and offer it to yourself. I want a meaningful job, close family and friends, and happy existence.

Check in again and take note of how you're feeling. Consider one individual or a group of persons to whom you wish to convey loving-kindness; imagine them seated or standing in front of you. Feel and sense them.

"I wish them peace and happiness. Wishing them a life free of fear, worry, and tension. Be concerned, be sad. I wish them happiness and joy. Wellbeing."

Allow this loving-kindness to spread. Allow it to expand and touch everyone you want this sensation to touch right now, in all directions. These might be folks you know or people you don't know. People with whom you have disagreements. People you adore without condition. Imagine this emotion contracting and extending, filling every animal or human it comes into contact with loving love. Everyone has changed.

You may imagine that everyone and everything is serene, pleasant, and at ease. Take a big breath in and open your eyes when you're ready.

Getting Rid of Negative Energy

We live in a world of twos, as was intended. There is right and wrong, and good and bad. The yin and yang idea exists both within and outside the body. The earth's plane is such an excellent classroom for soul development. We wouldn't have development, diversity, joy, or grief if there weren't a duality.

This implies that the energies and individuals we encounter teach us lessons we require while on our journey here. This might just be a reference to knowing how to cleanse, defend, and work with bad energy. It's easy to compare it to a video game.

During times of transition and severe stress, everyone might experience the effects of lesser energies. We occasionally absorb, accept, or attract lesser energy from those around us. All of this is part of the game, and these experiences will help us grow as souls and persons.

Here are some indicators that negative energy has taken hold of you:

- You may experience lost calls or static on your phone when chatting with someone in an area where you have a solid connection.
- You may feel depressed even though you have never been diagnosed with depression.
- You can't get into your bank or other online accounts because you keep getting an error message despite a robust internet connection.
- You become weary quickly and feel the need for a nap despite having slept well the night before.
- You refuse to help yourself, such as eating, even when hungry.
- You have a sore throat and flu-like symptoms.
- You misplace your wallet or keys, get your belongings stolen, or lock your keys in the car.

- Your email did not reach the target recipient, and you are then chastised for not contacting them.

- Your mind begins to race with bad memories of something or someone from your past. You try your hardest to shrug them off, but they adhere to you like glue.

- Your conduct becomes anti-self-love, such as spending too much money on useless items, especially if you don't have the money. This is crucial if this isn't your usual persona.

Because there are infinite possibilities, we must detect and observe these patterns because they are individualized. It might take you years to realize what is going on when you are influenced by bad energy. If you have a mixture of these in one day or a short period, it might help you recognize what is happening. As you begin to tune into your consciousness, it will become clearer.

When you discover you've picked up bad energies, there are various strategies you may utilize alone or in combination to assist rid your energy field, body, and mind of this negativity. Even if it was accidental, the opposite is true.

There are numerous individuals on the globe. Everyone has their interests and purposes. Some are favorable, while others are unfavorable. Others, on the other hand, choose to embrace negativity wholeheartedly.

It is impossible to exclude all bad people from your life. They might be coworkers or family members.

It is also impossible to alter these folks. This puts you in a difficult position, especially if you are a sensitive empath. There is hope; you can get out of that situation by improving yourself rather than changing others.

Methods for Getting Rid of Negativity

Declare that you are releasing this energy: Declaring your intentions aloud has tremendous power. This little act transforms them into genuine people. Make them a reality rather than just a notion. Begin by stating it out after you've determined that all the bad energy around you is enough and want to lessen it. You are not required to inform anybody. Simply put it out there and let your voice return to your ears. Take your intention and go forward to make it a reality.

- **Yawn:** Go ahead and do it. Many people believe that yawning is a symptom of dissatisfaction or boredom, yet it clears the body of unneeded energy. This should come as no surprise, given that breathing may help with anxiety. Yawning is just a strong, purposeful breath.

- **Smudge:** You spent the weekend with a nasty individual, and your home now seems heavy with bad energy. You may feel as if you have brought too much tension from work home. In any case, a smear may be necessary. White sage has been used in cleansing ceremonies to expel unwelcome spirits and energies for hundreds of years.

- **Say a Mantra:** This takes the declaration of your goal a step further by allowing you to command the bad energy out.

- I, (say your name), do not permit any non-physical or living person to enter my body, energy field, spirit, soul, or mind for any reason other than love.

- I violate any agreements, promises, or contracts that I may have mistakenly signed in any dimension, place, or time that would limit the expression of my joyous nature.

- I violate all agreements beginning with this now and continuing backward through all of my prior experiences and ahead till the end of time.

- I command that these persons and energies leave this location immediately! You no longer have authority over me. I want protection from these energies, so they do not return to my energy field. I create a luminous barrier around myself with my goal and free choice. I appreciate that it has been completed.

- Repeat this chant as many times as necessary.

- **Laugh:** Laughter is said to be the best medicine for a reason. It causes a shift in your body that increases positive energy while decreasing tension and discomfort. It may feel strange to laugh at nothing. Simply do it. Your chuckle will be real in a matter of minutes.

- **Dance:** When you dance, your brain releases endorphins. This generates a positive energy environment around you. It also discusses the universe. Joy is a high-vibrational state. This elevates you to a level that negativity cannot reach.

- **Acquire a Himalayan Salt Lamp:** A Himalayan salt lamp cleans the air around it and increases good energy. It generates negative ions that attract positive ions and emit negativity. It may appear counter-intuitive, but the effects are fantastic. There are several types of salt lamps.

- **Change Your Karma:** When confronted with bad energy, you may be inclined to return it in love. This achieves nothing. It will set you behind and lead you to use more energy. Perform acts of compassion. Assist someone less fortunate. Donate to your chosen charity. Participate in a food pantry volunteer program. These actions will eliminate bad energy and increase your karma.

- **Create a Negative Collector:** Set a glass of water on a table or light a candle. Declare your intention to channel all negative energy into the water or flame while staring at it. This will also alleviate physical and emotional issues.

- **Spend Time with Someone Special:** If you are in a relationship, sex can help you get rid of bad energy and replace it with positive energy. When two people have sex, other things happen, such as blood pressure reduction, immune system increase, and stress release.

- **Plants:** are an excellent way to filter out bad energy. Put it on in every room where you spend time. Another wonderful cleanser is to open the windows and let the sunlight through.

- **Salt:** Apply salt to your carpeting. Allow it to settle for about an hour before vacuuming. The salt naturally absorbs negative energy. You may also place salt bowls in the corners of each area. Allow it to rest for a few hours before removing it.

- **Claim the Space:** If your space is overrun with other people's belongings, stroll around and claim it. Once you've implanted positive energy, any bad energy that lingers will be unable to stay.

- **Room Spray:** Create a room spray using essential oils to remove bad energy. Patchouli, frankincense, lavender, and rose are the finest to utilize. This will also work on individuals. Simply sprinkle yourself softly.

- High-frequency music: Listening to music with high vibrations will significantly impact. We all know that music affects our energy levels. It works in the same way for spaces.

- **Declutter Your Office or House**: Negative energy is trapped in old objects. Documents, periodicals, newspapers, and outdated garments must be discarded. You should clean your residence. Do not simply vacuum and wash the dishes. Laundry, walls, curtains, and carpets should all be cleaned. Allow fresh air to enter by opening the windows. Do your business or house a happy atmosphere, and all bad energy will go.

- **Black Tourmaline:** This crystal is capable of dispelling negative energy. This crystal does not require clearing in the same way other crystals do. This can also work for humans. When traveling, simply place it in your handbag or pocket. It is beneficial for persons who are sensitive to electricity and require protection.

- **Change Your Thinking:** Get rid of your negative ideas. Don't let little issues disturb you. Don't judge or criticize others and try not to whine. You should love yourself more. You must forgive yourself. Nobody is without flaws. Don't focus on flaws or faults. Use positive affirmations regularly to help you change your negative ideas into good ones. Motivational and inspirational quotations do the same goal. Maintain a gratitude notebook. Spend a few minutes each day writing down why you are grateful. Don't act like a victim. Take charge of your life because you made it. Stop blaming others and start making changes in your own life.

- **Put Your Anxieties on Paper:** Make a list of everything that bothers you. It may appear large, but when you see it on paper, you will realize that it isn't and that you can manage it. This is to capture the bad energy within you and record it on paper. Make this list as long as possible. Try to write down all of your negative ideas. Every tense thought you're experiencing. Then throw away the paper. It should be discarded or burned.

- **Take a Bath:** A hot shower or bath might help you feel more energized. This is extremely simple. To unwind and relax, soak for 20 to 30 minutes. You may also enhance your bath with sea salt or fragrant oils. Salt baths are an excellent technique to purify your aura and boost your vigor and health.

- **Mediate:** Mediation boosts serotonin levels, which improves behavior and mood. It reduces anxiety and aids in attaining peace of mind and clarity. It will aid in healing your energy system and maintaining a bright energy field. Choose a tranquil setting. Clear your thoughts by lying or sitting comfortably. Meditation isn't difficult.

- **Visualize:** If you are concerned about something, imagine a good result. Visualize the end outcome in your head so you won't have to worry about it. Consider how it will make you feel and hold onto that sensation for as long as possible. Imagine a joyful dream if you have nothing to worry about but still feel down.

- **Work It Out:** When nothing else works, and you're still unhappy or furious, the greatest thing you can do is sweat it out. Exercise is an excellent approach to deal with worry, despair, and stress. Whatever you choose to do, whether it's tennis, walking, swimming, lifting weights, yoga, or jogging, a good workout may help you clear your mind of negative ideas.

CHAPTER 22: BREATHING TECHNIQUES & WAYS TO INCREASE CLAIRVOYANCE

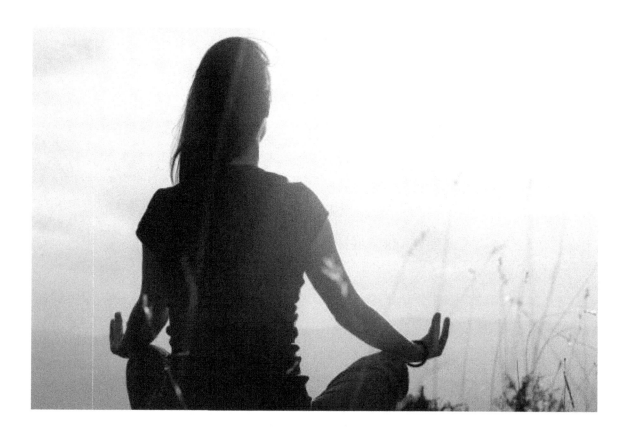

The Third Eye, often known as the sixth sense, is present in every one of us. Unfortunately, few people utilize it since they are unsure what to make of it. Learning how to activate or use the Third Eye is a huge accomplishment for anyone, and luckily, it is something that can be learned.

Breathing Techniques to Activate the Third Eye

It is critical first to identify the location of what you are attempting to activate. The Third Eye is located between the face, skull, and brain. It is critical to gain access to the Third Eye to activate it more easily. The best method to go there is to focus your attention in that direction, eyes closed and calm, and with a relaxed face. The head should be relaxed to the point that there are no stiff head muscles. Allow the head and face to fall so that your entire concentration is on where the Third Eye is located. You will become sidetracked, but there is a method around this by attempting to gather your photos. It is critical to visualize a certain subject or location where you will focus all of your imagination. You may imagine a little dot and focus all of your thoughts on it, working hard to ensure that you concentrate on that place. Allow no other ideas to distract you from your center of attention during that period of concentration. When you've gathered all of your ideas in one place, you're ready to focus even with your eyes wide open.

When you feel completely at peace and have made touch with your Third Eye, you may begin to increase your visualization. Begin cautiously, and don't put too much pressure on yourself to achieve the top when you aren't ready. Take your time visualizing whatever you want to deal with, don't be frightened if it takes a long time, and be patient yet sure. It is critical not to forget to have fun. Relax at each level of visualization; tensing up will simply distract you more. Attempt to reach the Third Eye with your eyes open, picturing the procedure, the travel, and how you truly feel connected to it. The mind is also located in the third region and aids in relaxing the eyes and brain. When the eyes and brain relax, the Third Eye gets stronger and easier to interpret. We also allow the sun's warmth to enter our bodies, freshening up the entire system and providing new energy levels. If the procedure becomes uncomfortable and even painful to your head, it is best to relax or let go, and you can always do it again when you are calmer.

People frequently make the mistake of trying to elevate their eyeballs to glimpse the Third Eye while still in visualization. The proper approach is to relax the eyes and let them remain in their regular position. Allow the eyes to rest in their sockets as you concentrate on your visualization of the Third Eye. Allow the neck to move slightly higher by elevating your head slightly. Take a deep breath and relax your face, neck, and shoulders once you are certain you are in this posture. Resting the eyes is one of the little hurdles you will face during the procedure to determine if you are doing it correctly. Imitate the sun's movement as it sets, and your eyes will immediately relax. You will begin to comprehend unexplainable knowledge when you can relax your bodily muscles. The exercise is critical because it serves as a link between a person, the heavens, and even the earth. There will also be a strong flow of energy throughout your body.

Having Third-Eye Sensation

Activating the Third Eye should not be rushed. It should be a progressive procedure in which you should not exert any pressure on yourself but instead inhale and give yourself time. Relaxing is a wonderful method to develop the imagery required in the Third Eye. If you can't relax naturally, take a break before beginning the meditation practice. Allow yourself to prepare for the meditation mentally you will undertake during that pause. Allow your mind to sense the energy to move through so that it will be simpler when you start. This will enable the Third Eye to become aware of what will happen, and the Third Eye will bring clarity. Reopening the Third Eye should not be a forced procedure; it should happen organically, so one should take their time. It takes years of training to complete the process; it does not happen overnight. Physical exercise, as well as mental preparation for a serene frame of mind, are required. Many individuals seek a quick procedure so that they may gain some form of enlightenment on numerous topics that they don't seem to understand. However, the fact is that the process is more psychological than physical, and the time it takes to achieve it varies depending on the individual.

The Third Eye is a fantastic approach to achieve internal tranquility and make someone more optimistic in their perception of things. You can either energize or soothe someone's spirit, depending on your energy. What spirit do you call upon when confronted with danger or adversity? If you react angrily or sorrowfully, you are elevating the spirit. However, when you allow yourself to be peaceful and relaxed in your mind, you quiet your soul because you are at peace with yourself.

Another lesson in what spirits we summon for ourselves comes from the thoughts we attract. What emotions do you expose yourself to regularly as a person? You are more prone to get depressed if you allow yourself to have unpleasant thoughts such as anger, despair, and discouragement regularly. You are instilling a low spirit inside yourself that only you can extinguish. A low spirit instills a sense of pessimism and sorrow and a weakened immune system in someone. This is why it is critical always to convey optimism to your brain rather than fostering negative thoughts. Positivity offers the body hope and power to battle on, regardless of how bad the circumstance is. It strengthens the body and keeps it healthy in general since that is the signal received from the body. Anyone can shift from negativity to positive; all you have to do is whisper and envision optimism anytime you want to give up. This will eventually stick, and you will be happy as a result.

When you use your eyes as the medium, you will be able to visualize. A passionate spirit is great; it gives you the strength to battle and face challenges you would never have imagined. That is the type of powerful energy you want to bring with you, more like a lion that has located its prey and is about to attack. Take a deep breath and gently exhale while you are in this state of intensity. This will give you a sensation of peace that will practically shake your body; your entire being will feel as if you were born anew. However, when you are in despair and feel defeated, it is good to seek support. You will not always be in command; no one is so powerful to manage problems all of the time. You don't want to be in denial about your sentiments since that's much worse than discussing them. However, if you dare to attempt, use the breathing approach to do the positive thought exercise. Some emotions are easily combated by breathing in and allowing positivity energy to flow. Breathe out all of the negativity that is trying to build up inside of you. Sometimes you feel so low that you don't want to use the little power, but you can't let your emotions prevail. You must seek out encouragement to help you overcome your poor moods.

The key to overcoming any level of mediocrity is to practice. Doing the workout regardless since not doing so will put you in a worse predicament. As you continue to practice, you will eventually be able to bring yourself out of the depressive condition, and you will be able to deal with it. You should execute the exercise more frequently, especially when you are not experiencing any difficulties. Practicing in the proper mental state prepares the mind for the days ahead. It also aids in the development of a persistent attitude of positivity so that difficult experiences do not rapidly unsettle you. When you cultivate optimism and are confronted with a negative event, the positivity within you will fight for you.

The Breathing Cycle

The first step is to breathe normally without straining anything. Pay attention to your breathing rhythm to better understand it. When you're confident, you've mastered the rhythm, attempt to regulate into little breaths. Smaller than your regular breathing pattern.

Second, you must take many deep breaths. Allow your breaths to be so deep that you can feel them inside you; you will feel as if you are being consumed. Deep breathing should be done via the nose and exhaled through the mouth. Allow this to continue for a time, making sure you are aware of every breath.

Finally, one should take rapid yet deep breaths for a few seconds. This is an attempt to reduce the air trapped in the lungs and belly. The breath inhaled should be retained inside for a few seconds before delicately exhaling it.

By doing this at least once a day, you will gain a sense of serenity that will progressively relax your body and mind, leading to the opening of your Third Eye. Grounding oneself is sometimes the only way to achieve a happy attitude. Taking grounding pauses to tackle a problem. Finally, you may require a bit longer than a day to employ multiple tactics over an emotion. Take your time inhaling since the Third Eye appears after the breathing procedure. The Third Eye will strengthen your intuition so that when you start to feel low, you will be able to stop yourself before it becomes serious and beyond your control. Third eye intuition can assist you in predicting scenarios that are likely to affect your moods and emotions. As a result, you will find yourself avoiding these circumstances more frequently. The Third Eye also promotes tranquility, which will become a personality feature while dealing with any situation. There is also knowledge associated with the Third Eye, which will provide you with sound judgment on matters. You might have responded to things with hate if you hadn't had Third Eye knowledge, but now you're cool as a cucumber. You must remember what you are attempting to accomplish with the breathing exercise. Concentrate on it so that you don't wind up doing anything more than breathing and expelling air. Remember to stick to the routine as much as possible until it becomes a habit. Sometimes our most intense negative emotions are buried deep within us, and the only way to let them go is to exhale them.

Steps to Increase Your Clairvoyance

Clairvoyance is a vital psychic skill that implies seeing clearly. The ability will provide you access to your soul's wisdom and the knowledge of all other souls in the world. This includes both former souls and those that have not yet manifested. It sounds nice, but there are some things to consider. Practicing these tactics daily can improve your skills. You may draw a parallel between learning a new language and working out. You will take your time, and you must put your energy into the practices to build your talents over time. Be nice and tolerant to yourself and avoid becoming frustrated if you find you aren't making any progress. Continue to try, and it will all work out in the end.

You should do the following to strengthen your clairvoyant abilities:

Step 1: Release and Unblock Your Clairvoyant Fears

You may encounter clairvoyant manifestation in your life in one form or another. You may have even blocked it without realizing it. The first step is to unblock and release the concerns building up in you about the wonderful talent.

Find a quiet spot and concentrate on your breathing to attempt to pinpoint the root of your anxiety. Do not be concerned about going off the deep end or experiencing psychic occurrences. Understand the distinction between psychotic and psychic episodes. Don't worry about what other people may say or think when they understand you have this priceless talent. You would believe that turning it off is a good way to respond, but that is not the case. You must discover a technique to release your fear and an affirmation to repeat regularly. Repeat that remark as many times as you can until your concern is gone.

Step 2: Maintain Your Concentration on the Third Eye

When you have completed the first step, it is time to begin the second phase: focusing on your Third Eye. The Third Eye chakra is located right above the brows. It is in charge of visual talents such as perceiving visions, symbols, and flashes.

Close your eyes and focus your attention on the space between your brows. You must assume that it has a horizontal-oval form and is located between your eyes. Take note of whether the Third Eye lid is opening or shutting. If it is closed, you must beg it to open and repeat until it does so. When your Third Eye opens, you will sense the love and a warm flow in your body. It will be so because you are experiencing an encounter with the blocked portion of yourself.

It's understandable if you can't envision your Third Eye on the first try. You must continue to do so, and with time, you will succeed. You must massage the Third Eye to activate and awaken it. As the power of your powers grows, so will the power of your other senses.

Step 3: Strengthen Your Visual Imagination

When your Third Eye agrees to open, you will notice shimmering lights, dots, images, and floating shadows. The pictures can take many shapes and hues. It may be in either black and white or full color. They may move or not, and they can have life or appear like a cartoon.

The initial image you are likely to view may be blurry and hazy. Before using your clairvoyant gift, you must first improve your visual imagination. You will put that knowledge to use by answering some particular questions. You must improve your visual inventiveness, and you may ask for the picture to be clearer and brighter and develop in size and strength. You must ensure that you employ all of your power and purpose to make that request.

You have to imagine yourself standing in a flower garden or field. Assume you are standing and holding numerous balloons that are not all the same color. Continue to believe that you have released one of them as you watch it soar up into the sky. When the balloon has completely vanished, go on to the next one and use your imagination in the same way. You must repeat this process until you can tell when each balloon is no longer visible.

Step 4: Using Clairvoyance, Answer Specific Questions

You must practice answering questions using your talents once you believe you are ready. The inquiries should be specific and have a point of concentration. You must limit your queries to those not wide, as large questions will deplete your energy and provide no beneficial results. You must always ask precise and well-formulated questions. Instead of asking generic queries, be extremely clear about what you want.

Step 5: Examine Clairvoyant Images

The mental images will appear from time to time. Once you can see them, you must also be able to comprehend and interpret them to make use of your visions. If you believe the pictures are illogical, you might ask the higher spirits silently or aloud for clarification. The higher senses will provide you with answers in the form of an emotion, sound, or thinking. You could think of them as hazy or random at first, but don't be concerned. It's natural, and you should trust yourself and the higher spirits. You may also ask the question again. The higher spirits will make certain that you receive the answer until you are satisfied that it is apparent.

Step 6: You Must Believe and Work with Faith

It is a critical step that will assist you in strengthening your clairvoyant abilities. You must believe and trust in what you see or hear. You must not diminish your abilities or dismiss them as a fantasy or a figment of your imagination. Wishful thinking and creativity can help you achieve many things, and you will be able to fully utilize your abilities. You will employ your clairvoyant power as a result, and you will appreciate life more and view things from a different perspective.

Step 7: Document Your Psychic Experiences

When you have completed all of the tasks in step 6, you are ready to go to step 7. You must keep a diary of your psychic encounters over some time. That will be a wonderful technique to assist you in furthering your development and understanding the psychic powers you possess. When you acknowledge such abilities, you will value the person you are becoming and will have the potential to grow in terms of strength.

It doesn't matter if you're acquiring claircognizance, clairaudience, clairvoyance, or clairsentience; you must document it. When you write it down, you will make it a habit to return to the notebook and read what is in it. You will discover how useful, genuine, and dependable your clairvoyant ability is. You will better understand your most dependable psychic and intrusive abilities. As a result, you will have greater power and strength to exercise control over yourself. You will realize the sort of life you are leading and the priceless treasure you own.

Step 8: Locate a Clairvoyant

Everyone has their way of looking at things. Having a new view on the situation from someone with similar abilities will help you respect yourself. You will realize that you are not the only one with such abilities, and your dread will go. Find someone with whom you can open up about your clairvoyant experiences, and it will be of great assistance to you. You will have the opportunity to learn from one another and discuss ideas from everyone's perspective. As a result, you will be able to assist and grow with one another. Knowing that you have someone to talk to if you become overwhelmed will make the journey more bearable.

Step 9: Meditate

If you wish to cultivate and enhance your psychic talent, you must meditate regularly. When you meditate, you will connect with your higher self and become more sensitive to intuitive teachings. Meditation will be extremely helpful in opening the Third Eye and increasing your mind's eye to visualize more.

Meditate with a specific goal in mind: to improve your clairvoyant abilities. You will be able to open and strengthen your Third Eye. You can go on a guided meditation or do the meditation yourself. It might be either a short one or the one you decide to go with, but it must be consistent. When you get guided meditation, you will be able to trust the visions that you are experiencing. You will believe that any visions you see are an important component of developing your clairvoyant powers.

While working to improve your clairvoyance, keep in mind that it is a similar sensation to daydreaming. To be effective, you must be patient while going through this procedure. It will take some time, and you have rehearsed everything to the finish, so if you fail along the way, you will have wasted your time and efforts. Because your time and energy are so valuable, you must exercise caution in how you spend them. Spending them isn't such a smart idea. When it comes to increasing your clairvoyant power, there are no shortcuts.

One individual will receive psychic energy more naturally than the other. Because no two people are alike, you should not be concerned if your gift is not stronger than the other person's. You have psychic strength that has nothing to do with curses or the dark side. It is a technique to strengthen your connection to your creator, and it will propel you to greater spiritual heights.

Allow your thoughts to relax and reflect on everything that has happened to you. You must relinquish control to God. Remove any negativity you may have before beginning your spiritual connection. Maintain a positive aura around yourself, and you will be able to eliminate negativity within you. This will serve as a safeguard, so there will be no roadblocks along the way. You may notice that the adventure becomes more enjoyable as you progress through it. You will notice that the closer you get to God and your spirituality, the clearer everything becomes.

CHAPTER 23: THINKING POSITIVELY

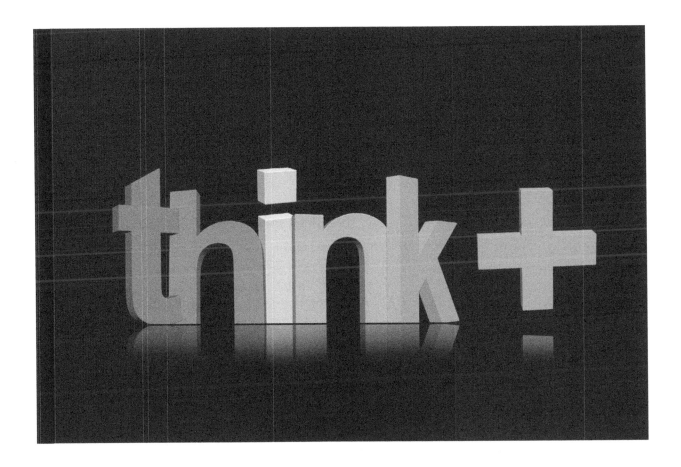

The laws of energy are a well-known natural force. We all know that we are more likely to get positive energy when we give out positive energy. Positive energy is not only what we put out there; it is also what we believe inwardly.

Let's start with what we say and how we act. We've all met a person or two in our lives who always speaks negative things and finds the worst in everything. What are your thoughts about the person? Would you sense a good or negative aura if you saw their aura? Would they have any radiance at all?

Is it common for that individual to have negative things happen to them? Is their fortune a little skewed? It's no surprise that they're pulling negative energy to themselves. On the other hand, if we look at what positive individuals tend to attract, spreading optimism brings about good energy and karma.

Is it possible to change the trajectory of our life just by thinking positively? Absolutely! We've discovered that thinking positively attracts nice things to you, but it also retrains your brain to think positively. On a personal level, thinking positively makes it simpler to complete activities and reach goals.

For example, if you want to graduate college and start a profession, having a bad attitude can hinder your progress and prevent you from starting. You're talking yourself out of even applying to universities because you're afraid you won't get admitted.

This fear and negativity will prevent you from living the life you desire. Replacing negative with positive ideas boosts your confidence, reinforcing the concept that you can achieve everything you set your mind to if you put out a genuine effort.

Take a few minutes off from reading. Simply keep track of the things going through your mind for 10 minutes. Consider how many of your ideas are pure and positive and how many are unsure, negative, or pessimistic. What precisely are you getting out of this? With hundreds of ideas racing through your mind every day, this adds to many negative energy being squandered.

It is now time to retrain your mind to think positively. The brain is an extraordinary organ, taking in and digesting information from the moment we breathe our first breath. The brain physically receives data from your eyes, ears, and other sense organs. The brain analyzes it as rapidly as possible to make sense of information.

Once a choice is made, a neural route from signal to comprehension is formed. When this signal is detected again, it may be processed swiftly to this unavoidable understanding. Consider touching your hand to a hot burner. You will establish a road to knowing that touching it causes pain, which you will never do again.

While this has obvious benefits in terms of physical danger, it does not work so well in other aspects of life. A potential boyfriend or girlfriend is rejecting that perceived threat. Because of the unpleasant experience, you learn not to take chances and talk to partners for fear of being rejected in the future. This impedes your life's growth.

The good news is that new routes can be constructed to replace existing ones. All that is required is awareness of your thoughts and the capacity to intentionally reroute those ideas to positive results. This method will need time, but the ultimate result will undoubtedly be worthwhile. Begin with these simple steps to create a more positive life for yourself.

Keep track of your thoughts every day. You can do this by committing to at least 10 minutes of thought monitoring. Take some time to jot down your thoughts for what they are.

Rework your thoughts. When you have a bad idea, concentrate on it and actively work to change it. For example, if you are caught in traffic, you may believe that you will never make it to work on time and have a poor day. Instead, consider what you can do to improve the situation. Can you phone work and inform them? Would this help to relieve the tension? Even if it doesn't, the circumstance is what it is, so why not enjoy it? Take in the environment around you, listen to your favorite music, and take some time to unwind. What you make of it is up to you.

Start your day with a good thought. If your day is dominated by negativity, the sound of your alarm clock sets the tone for the rest of the day. Before getting out of bed, turn on the light, take in your surroundings, and think about something nice to look forward to that day. Consider what you are grateful for, what exciting activity you have planned for today, or anything else to help you start the day off correctly.

CHAPTER 24: ENERGY HEALING

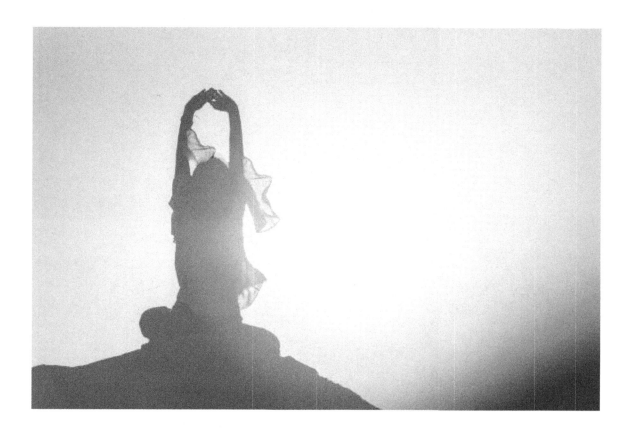

Like adopting a balanced diet, managing your inner energy necessitates some upkeep. The activities you choose to engage in, both physical and mental, impact the health of your inner energy, or chi as it is known in Eastern medicine. Energy healing does not involve a large investment of money or time, but it does necessitate some effort and, for beginners, the supervision of an experienced healer.

Let us start with the most basic mechanism of all: energy transmission. This directs the flow of energy around your body. Energy travels circularly throughout your body, but it may get obstructed, causing a buildup in certain areas while starving others. Consider this energy to be your blood rushing through your veins. If a blockage cannot be removed, it might produce catastrophic difficulties inside the system.

Energy transfer is a simple method that you may do every day to keep your energy flowing, and it is an excellent addition to your meditation practice. Thought and gentle touch may be used to flow energy through your body. The objective is to identify the location of the blockage so that you can target it. This might be a bodily symptom, such as shoulder soreness or a stomach ache. Simply sit motionlessly and softly lay your hands over the affected region.

For example, if your stomach is unhappy, softly lay your hands on your stomach. Consider how much energy is accumulating in your hands throughout your body, then imagine the energy flowing from your hands into your tummy, showering it with wellness.

It will take some practice to get a sense of the impacts of this strategy. It takes a lot of focus to capture that energy and appropriately disperse it. Seek the assistance of a professional if you are new to meditation and energy work. It is possible to perform energy work on another person, but you may need to draw energy from another individual to feel the effects.

A trained Reiki practitioner can assist you in discovering where your energy needs to be improved and help you reopen the doors of spiritual contact. Reiki is accessible and useful to everyone, including those dubious of its effectiveness. Energy is unconcerned with doubt and will continue to work regardless of belief.

Reiki is not a religion; thus, it is accessible to everyone. You do not need to believe in any religious parts of the practice, making it more of an open field, similar to massage treatment or acupuncture.

When engaging with a practitioner intimately, it is critical to trust and feel at ease with this individual. Some people you may not get along with, while others you may. Don't give up if your first Reiki treatment doesn't go as planned. Give the benefit of the doubt and try again or seek the services of another practitioner.

Acupuncture is another excellent method for removing energy blockages and restoring energy flow. Around 6000 BC, this old ritual began in China. Practitioners utilized sharpened animal bones instead of needles to target various pressure points across the body.

When you apply pressure and a skin prick to an area of concern, your body sends blood flow and energy to that region to repair it. This surge of energy clears the system, alleviating the symptoms. Acupuncture may treat almost any condition, from physical pain to mental distress.

Because acupuncture requires a clean, sterile atmosphere, it is best to get treatment from a qualified physician. Find someone with sufficient education and licensed by your local health agency. Because these needles have the potential to spread infections, having a practitioner who follows the guidelines and disposes of old needles is critical.

Moving your body is another excellent approach to release stored energy. We've known for a long time that there's a link between general activity and overall health. We think of a healthy person as someone who moves their body regularly. Starting or increasing a current exercise plan can significantly enhance energy flow and overall health.

Not all forms of exercise are equal. Many people mistake exercising only in some sections of their bodies while neglecting others. A walker, for example, may work their legs and heart, but their upper body remains entirely untested. A bodybuilder may concentrate on muscular mass but not on cardiovascular fitness. The majority of individuals concentrate too much on the workout and not enough on the stretching.

Furthermore, most exercises are not performed with optimal energy flow in mind. People focus on the work but not the goal, while the goal is to establish a channel of energy flow that delivers oxygen and blood to all sections of the body, including essential organs. Some workouts are more effective than others in this regard.

Yoga is a beautiful discipline that has gained popularity in the fitness industry over the last decade. There are several versions and classes available, each with its own beliefs about what is correct. None of them are incorrect; they are simply different. Some courses focus on the same set of postures, while others vary the practice frequently, while others focus mostly on meditation.

Find an approach that speaks to you by experimenting with numerous variations and determining what makes you feel your best. Yoga's instant effects are obvious. Those who practice describe sensations of exhilaration and lightness in their body immediately following practice and for the remainder of the day. The technique lowers tension, stretches your muscles, and shifts energy.

Yoga does need some fundamental physical strength and capacity, but it is also something that increases with practice. It is a terrific alternative if you are in excellent health and can move. Pose changes are also feasible if your movement is restricted.

Qigong and tai chi are both ancient disciplines that emphasize energy flow. If you saw someone doing either, it may remind you of karate or another martial art, but at a much slower speed. The hand and leg motions are similar to conventional techniques in a continuous slow-motion flow. It's quite a sight, and the stress release and physical exercise benefits linked with this practice improve energy flow.

Whatever energy therapy you practice, consistent participation in something that helps keep your energies balanced is essential in today's hectic environment. At any time, your energy might change in one direction or another. It is critical to identify this and make the appropriate modifications so that you may live your best life.

CHAPTER 25: PSYCHIC AWARENESS

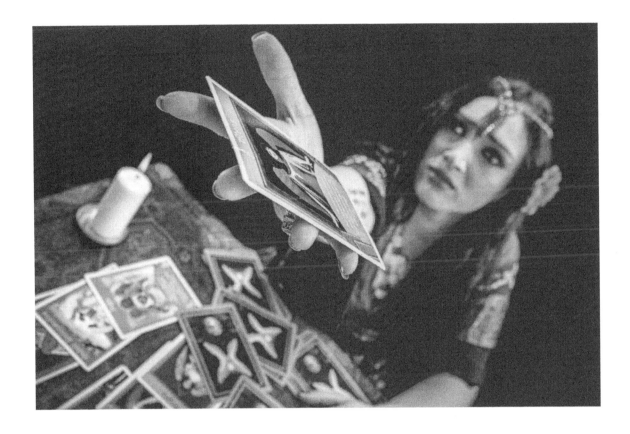

Psychic awareness is described as "awareness of human consciousness and the full power of the mind when applied to daily life." Psychic awareness is defined as the comprehension of the quiet spirit that dwells inside us and the power of our minds. This psychic awareness gives us access to our subconscious mind, allowing us to manage the many internal forces that impact our health, wellness, and interpersonal connections.

There are strategies to improve as well as increase your psychic awareness. The power of psychic awareness can be used in numerous aspects of our existence. Consider your brain to be a computer when considering psychic awareness. When a computer is disconnected, it may still be used, but its capabilities are severely restricted. However, when a computer is linked to the internet, it has an almost limitless number of activities that it may accomplish. When you activate your Third Eye, it's as if you're linking your brain to the spiritual powers of the cosmos (you then unlock endless possibilities and potential by utilization of your psychic awareness).

We've all heard the scientifically supported notion that humans only use about 10% of our brain's gray matter. Could the remaining untouched 90% have a lot to do with psychic awareness? By practicing psychic awareness techniques, such as those used to achieve Third Eye waking, we will be able to access and utilize the remaining 90% of our brains.

Tips for Increasing and Strengthening Your Psychic Awareness

- **Pray** – Whatever higher force you believe in, whatever religion you follow, ask that higher power to assist you in unlocking deeper psychic awareness.

- **Meditate** – Through meditation, we may disengage from the general din of life and instead develop a connection to a deeper awareness of our surroundings and inner selves. When you let go of preoccupying anxious thoughts, you will be able to accept your mind's natural sense of intuition more readily.

- **Journal** – Journaling is an excellent technique for being aware of the external stressors in your life that tend to fog your thoughts the most. Once you can recognize these stressors, you will be able to learn when to let go and continue with your Third Eye waking activities.

Heal Yourself by Using Your Mind

Good day and welcome. Thank you for joining me in this self-healing meditation today. This meditation was created to help anyone suffering from diseases, discomforts, or other bodily issues.

You will be directed to calm down throughout this meditation. You will speak with your body during this time, bestowing blessings, health, and love on it.

This meditation is designed to enhance self-love and cure ourselves. We look for answers to our life's issues in our immediate surroundings and beyond.

We often overlook the power to heal when it comes to our bodies. It's important to realize that you'll never be wiser than your body.

Doctors are vital in your recovery process, but they can only establish an atmosphere conducive to healing. True healing arises from inside you.

You are well aware that bad thoughts result in negative bodily manifestations. You should commit to listening to your body, nurturing it, and providing it with the self-care it demands.

Most disorders in our bodies are caused by imbalances such as too much fat, too much salt, too much resentment, too much stress, insufficient sleep, or insufficient tranquility.

Let us seek equilibrium and allow our bodies to heal during today's meditation. This meditation should be done regularly before going to bed or when you get up. Please choose a quiet location where you will not be interrupted.

Maintain a straight spine when you stand up. Maintain a comfortable posture with your palms facing up and make sure they do not contact your arms or legs. Make yourself at ease.

I appreciate you taking the time out of your busy schedule to read this. I'd like to connect with you and learn about your body's wonderful ways to repair itself.

It is critical to understand that you are both unconscious and conscious.

It is OK if your subconscious mind contains only good ideas.

To cure your body, you must accept some realities and become aware of the messages lurking in the shadows of your subconscious mind.

Please consider this suggestion: We are 95 percent unconscious and only 5% awake.

Please consider that your brain can process a large quantity of data in a second, but it can only be conscious of a limited portion of it.

Every single day, your body performs heavenly duties.

Every second of every day, it does some data to keep you alive when you chat, sleep, or drive.

You may not have given it much care in the past, but now is the moment to think about and respect this temple that houses your ideas, memories, childhood beliefs, and you as a person.

Allow your body to unwind. Concentrate on one portion at a time and relax.

Slowly take in and exhale. Take note of the sensations in your nostrils as you inhale and exhale.

Close your eyes and take a deep breath.

What sensations do you have as your breath enters and departs your body?

Allow yourself another deep breath and allow it to clear your system. Slowly exhale, releasing the tension in your body.

Allow your body to get heavy with each breath.

Allow your body to relax, beginning with the soles of your feet. Is there a tingling feeling in your hands? It should feel like you're treading on a fur rug. Feel the energy stroking your ankles as you relax your feet.

Feel it creep up to your knees. Can you feel it coursing up your upper legs?

Please don't fight it or attempt to stop it. Allow the energy to fill your entire system; feel it go to your hips, arms, and wrist.

Allow it to contact every area of your body and feel the effect. Allow it to migrate to your fingers. Do they feel comfortable? Allow it to rise to your collarbone, nose, eyes, and cheeks.

Do you sense the energy's power? Allow it to run its course.

Your eyelids should be relaxed. Allow them to feel heavy before relaxing.

Relax your ears and forehead by letting your brows relax. Take note of the energy that flows through them.

Your brow should be relaxed. Does it have a cool and calm vibe about it?

Extend your relaxation to the top of your head. You should now feel tranquil since you have relaxed your entire body. Can you feel the calm enveloping you from head to toe?

Allow your spine to unwind. Begin from the back of your head and work your way down to your tailbone. Feel your muscles relax.

Feel all of your back muscles release and relax totally. Allow calmness to spread throughout your body. Use that energy to quench your system's hunger.

Take a deep breath and hold it for a few seconds. Relax all of your muscles before slowly exhaling via your mouth or nose. Do you notice your limbs becoming heavy and then relaxing?

Take another deep breath and let your body relax.

Allow it to flow out with the little tension lodged in your muscles.

Continue to breathe gently and evenly. Examine your body for any leftover tightness. Is there any strain anywhere? Take your stress-relieving energy there. Allow it to flow in that place, carrying the tension with it.

Consider the air you breathe to be cleaner. Consider how it may relieve all of your body's tension. Assume that the air you breathe contains relaxing energy. Visualize the stress dissipating with each breath you take.

Can you feel how relaxed and tranquil your body is? Now take a few moments to relish the sensation.

(Pause)

Concentrate your attention on your body and consider the area that needs healing.

Think about your current state of being. Consider the bodily ailment that is bothering you. It makes no difference whether it is pain, an injury, a disease, or a diagnosis. Consider whatever it is. Consider the problem for which you wish to find a solution.

Concentrate your attention on the exact area where your problem is located.

Consider your issue to be darkness and your recovery to be a brilliant light. Visualize brilliant light streaming from your head to your toes. Allow your body to flow completely.

Now, aim it at your darkness.

Your body is capable of self-healing. Notice how the brilliant light boosts your immune system, giving you strength, eradicating bacteria and toxins, and thoroughly cleaning your system.

Consider the bright light flowing, caressing, and whirling over the blackness in the affected area of the body.

Can you see the shards of darkness vanishing from your system? As you breathe, allow them to escape.

Breathe in good health, serenity, and healing, and exhale stress, tension, illness, and any other issues in your system.

Allow the dazzling light to float over the darkness while it works its spell. Take note of how the blackness is shrinking and growing lighter. The intense light carries everything detrimental to your body.

Consider your immune system starting up and the cells moving to their proper locations. They are carrying out their responsibilities to heal your body.

Visualize a brilliant light coursing through your body. Feel your body filling up with relaxing sensations. Imagine your diseased body parts repairing and shrinking. Imagine it lightening up, relaxing, and taking away all the pain and discomfort—healing.

Allow your body to repair itself.

Breathe in the cleaner and expel any garbage.

Allow your body to relax while you breathe in and out any undesired substances in the system. Have faith in your body's ability to recover. Feel the serenity.

(Pause)

Observe your body feeling light as if it has been unburdened.

Feel more room in your mind and body.

Feel how light your limbs are.

Take note of the wonderful contentment that is coursing through your body.

It is now time to return to our typical degree of alertness.

Feel your mind and body becoming more conscious of your surroundings.

Slowly deepen your breath while you focus your attention on your surroundings.

Do you have a sense of your heartbeat?

Pay attention to any nearby voice.

What voices do you hear on the other end?

You have reasserted your body's ability to heal.

You've gotten close to the truth about your self-healing.

You've made a permanent alteration in your path.

Accept the modification. Recognize that you have become your healer.

I'm going to count to five. You'll be back to your regular level of awareness by the time I get to five.

1

2

3

4

5

Welcome back.

You'll be ready to start your day in a few minutes. You will have more energy and a lighter heart.

Thank you for practicing with me, and I hope you enjoy your newfound energy and revitalized physique. Have a wonderful day ahead of you.

CHAPTER 26: ENHANCED PSYCHIC ABILITIES

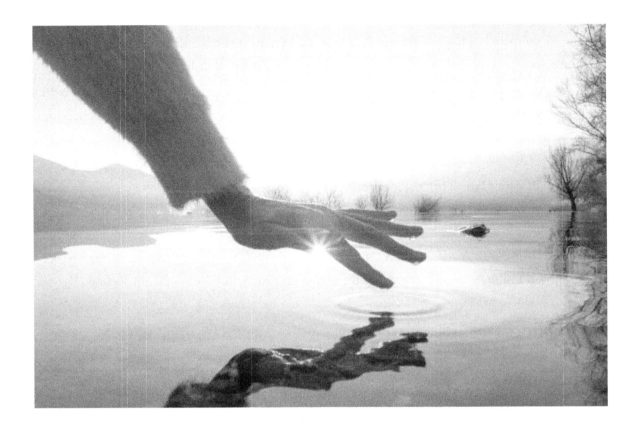

Third Eye awakening improves several psychic abilities, the most common of which are increased learning ability, increased creativity, clairvoyance (psychic vision), clairaudience (psychic hearing), clairsentience (psychic feeling), increased intuition, and the ability to see or sense the auras of others. The Third Eye, also known as the sixth chakra, is most well-known for its enhanced perception and vision. The Third Eye broadens cosmic consciousness and fosters a sense of connectedness to the cosmos.

One may question why it is significant or why they should be interested in improving their psychic talents. The answer is simple: psychic powers assist us in avoiding unpleasantness or unneeded suffering in our lives. These diverse psychic skills may be used to discern which route in life should be chosen to achieve success and make the best judgments possible. Psychic powers are not a talent that only a few people have; everyone has some psychic ability and can enhance it.

Some ways for developing and increasing your psychic skills (other than meditation, of course) are put in a list for you below:

- **Practice Psychometry:** Comparable to intuition, practicing psychometry is a wonderful technique to improve your present psychic talents. When you practice psychometry, you are attempting to read the energy of an inanimate item. Close your eyes and grip an object firmly in your palm (ideally one made of metal). Concentrate all of your attention on the thing in your hand and try to utilize your intuition to intuit facts about the object's owner.

- **Work with Zener Cards:** Zener cards are a terrific tool for dramatically improving your psychic talents. To utilize Zener cards, ask a buddy to select a card and memorize it (without displaying or telling you which card they are holding). Then request that they try to mentally project the card picture to you as you utilize your psychic talents to receive the card's image telepathically.

- **Go to an Antique Store:** Antique stores are full of older objects with years of history behind them. Simply being in a setting with many historical connections can improve your psychic talents. Visit an antique store in your region and use your natural intuition to see what you feel by being surrounded in this setting.

- **Telepathy Phone Call:** This exercise may be fun once your psychic talents are strong enough to accomplish them effectively. Relax and focus all of your energy on a select buddy, using only your intellect and psychic abilities. Concentrate on requesting this specific person to call you within the next 24 hours in your mind. After you've felt you've focused your energies on this work, wait to see whether your friend's intuition was able to pick up the signal and call you based on a gut feeling.

Spiritual Healing

It is difficult to have a spirit made up of energy. Like the energy in your home, the electricity might go out. While your lights may flicker and your TV show may be halted briefly, a spiritual outage is far more devastating. If your spirit is extinguished, the remainder of your life becomes extremely hard to live since you no longer have your guide. The good news is that every spirit has a lit flame, no matter how dim.

Spiritual illumination can be suffocated by everyday existence. We all wind up in the circumstances we don't want to be in, do jobs we don't want to do to make ends meet, or hang around with people who are a poor influence and don't respect us. Our inner self dims when we do or say things not in line with our spiritual nature.

It is quite simple to go down this road. Our culture has taught us to sit, be quiet, and do what we are told. While we are learning several things simultaneously, we are not always living up to our genuine spiritual potential, which has no boundaries and is not constrained by society's rules.

We must learn to live within the framework we are given while still charting the course that will lead us to true happiness. To be more explicit, the fundamental structure would be something along the lines of "respect others, don't damage anyone, and pay your taxes." The rest is up to you. That is rather lenient, allowing your spirit full reign over everything else. Despite this, the majority of us do not. We never attain our full potential because we live in a governed world. We don't want to annoy anyone by doing our own thing, as nice youngsters.

A broken spirit influences everything you do. For example, you may have recently ended a horrible relationship. It might be a friend, spouse, or coworker. This individual may have taken advantage of you by requesting favors with no reciprocation, being mentally manipulative, etc. As a result, the body and intellect are estranged from the soul. This relationship would have terminated long ago if your spirit had any say in the matter.

As a result, there is a general lack of liveliness. You may have been unhappy or nervous, sacrificing your own needs to meet the needs of others. Over time, this stress can have physical consequences, resulting in health issues such as persistent colds and flu due to a weakened immune system. Because your body is depleted of energy, you may have a general sense of drowsiness. You may even develop major illnesses such as heart disease or autoimmune disorders, as stress is often the root cause.

Now that this scenario has been addressed, it is time to reestablish your relationship, whether by your will or theirs. There are several tools available to help us reconnect with our inner selves, and it is worthwhile to focus on. Your life will return to you once you reconnect with your inner self. You will feel enthusiastic, driven, and capable if you are on the correct track. Your health may improve as a result of making better health-related decisions. You will no longer require food, drink, cigarettes, or your preferred crutch to cope with stress.

Spiritual healing manifests itself in a variety of ways. There are many skilled healers available that can help you shift your energy and get back on track. If you are unsure where to begin, it may be useful to consult with a healer to gain your bearings and figure out where to go from here. With their assistance, you may balance your inner energy and have those energy systems aligned and flowing properly. Their advice can provide you with the comfort you require to go forward with your life and return to normalcy.

If you are more confident in your abilities, attempt some self-care at home. Learning skills like Reiki and meditation on your own may be simple and quite rewarding. Many people feel better at ease making this trip alone, without the involvement of others. This is a personal choice, and because it is their want, they will be phenomenally successful if they take steps alone.

If you believe your only physical difficulties, don't rule out spiritual healing. For example, if you believe you have gotten diabetes or high blood pressure out of nowhere, you have a lot of work to do. Sure, you don't exercise, and your diet has been abysmal recently, but spiritual healing can get to the bottom of why you made those terrible choices in the first place. No one in their right mind (or soul) would desire to hurt their body; stress and other life concerns are typically the cause.

While you should still consult a medical doctor to handle these issues, reconnecting with your soul, altering things in your life that you are dissatisfied with, and resuming your spiritual journey will change everything. Consider this: If everything were going well at work, you had a plethora of wonderful family and friends, and you were happy, wouldn't it be simpler to eat healthier and exercise? The stress of negative relationships and events causes a chain reaction of negativity that results in physical stress symptoms.

Spiritual healing is completely free. It's simple, and it's what your body craves. It is aware that it should be intricately connected with the spirit, yet our minds fool us into believing that we have it all figured out on our own. You have to pay attention to the very loud, very evident signals our spiritual nature sends us. The stress we experience, the illnesses we get, and the gut emotions we ignore are signs from our spirit that we have wandered from our path. They are means of communicating with us to find our way back to the right road.

Everything falls into place once we get back on track and stop struggling against the energy of the cosmos. If you feel you can't do anything right, it's your spirit speaking to you, telling you that it's time to quit what you're doing and alter your path. This might be as easy as being kinder to others, letting others go first in traffic congestion, being friendlier to coworkers, or even uprooting your entire life and starting anew. Allow things to go, minimize your angst, and allow some optimism. Start with the road rage and work your way up from there. Bringing in positive energy rather than negative energy can nourish your spirit and improve your entire existence. It all starts with a single modest step.

Spiritual Healing Power

The process may begin once you've identified a spiritual healing path. This may be a long and winding journey with many twists and turns. You may not know where you are going, but you must trust your intuition and recognize that your spirit is connected to universal nature. Energy is quite simple; it flows via the path with the least amount of resistance. It knows where it's headed and can see the quickest route there. Your energy level is the same. If you listen and follow it, you will wind up precisely where you should be. That conclusion may surprise you.

If you're not sure about this entire thing yet, learn from a few folks who take daily measures to connect with their inner self and discover direction. Many others have gone before you, gotten to know their inner selves, and led better lives. Remember, the only endpoint is our death. Thus, we must continue to listen. It is never too late to begin your journey toward wellness and a higher quality of life.

As an example, consider Amy. Amy is the successful company owner's daughter, and she grew up working at her father's restaurant. As the company flourished, it became a gag in the family that Amy would someday take over the company when her father retired. Amy grimaced when this was brought up at the ripe old age of seventeen. She felt uneasy with the concept, but she couldn't put her finger on why. She enjoyed serving tables with her sisters and relatives at the restaurant.

Amy decided to take some business management classes at college in the hopes of finding some drive to take over the restaurant. When she graduated, her father recruited her to operate the restaurant while he retired. It had always been his ambition to retire early and live off the proceeds of his successful enterprise. Amy desired the same thing for him.

Amy marries and has a few children throughout the years. Her time is primarily spent at the restaurant, where she does the finances, orders supplies, and does her best to manage. She gained weight throughout the years, eating the diner-style food that surrounded her and doing nothing to exercise the magnificent physique that this world had put together for her. Because she is exhausted and overworked, she becomes grumpy and unapproachable. Her employee turnover rises as waiters and chefs struggle to deal with her demeanor. She divorces after many years of tense silence in her marriage with her spouse.

Amy is at a crossroads. She is now in her forties and wonders what happened to her life. Her mind was filled with ideas of what she might have done to be happy, slimmer, and keep her marriage together – all useless ideas because the past cannot be altered.

Amy is presented with some spare time because the kids spend the weekends with their father. She starts to think and listen. She finds herself lured to information about stress management and relaxation on the internet. She stumbles upon one regarding spiritual healing that piques her attention. The thought of meditation and listening to her inner self is quite appealing, and her soul wanted her to see it.

She starts making time to meditate every day. She begins slowly, with only a few mindful thoughts every day and a little recording of her emotions. As she begins to feel her tension dissipate, she looks into other choices, including seeing a professional healer for advice. As soon as she walks into the restaurant, she notices how defeated she is. Just thinking about it has sapped her spirit.

She pays attention to these warning flags and finally decides to exit the firm. As she arrives at this knowledge, there is no grand discovery, no pyrotechnics. In reality, she has no notion what she would do instead, other than that managing the firm is no longer functioning. She feels terrified, frightened, and unsure of what to do with this discovery.

She gradually develops the courage to approach her father about stepping down. He reluctantly agrees but understands that his presence progressively kills her physically and emotionally.

Amy's spiritual recovery is being aided by frequent meditation and mindfulness practice. While she is interested in various subjects, she has always been drawn to the marketing aspect of the restaurant industry. She has always liked creating weekly specials and maintaining an internet presence. This was a creative outlet for her, and her astute marketing talents kept the company afloat for years.

She is currently obtaining a marketing degree, improving her connections with her children, and living a more purposeful life. She began exercising after noticing her physique deteriorating and realizing it was an unhealthy vehicle for the growing soul within.

Amy is still a work in progress, but she has returned to her original path by surrendering to the natural flow. Sure, she never anticipated being a middle-aged, divorced mother in college. Still, she is happier than she ever was at the restaurant, and her newfound zest for life is more than enough to propel her forward to the next adventure.

Amy's experience is not unusual, but it is unique to her. We've all heard the stories of how people on the verge of bankruptcy turn their fortunes around and become billionaires. Sure, your spirit will bring you there, but it isn't concerned about money. The earlier you recognize this, the better. Our spiritual achievements are assessed in terms of happiness, satisfaction, love, and vitality, not in terms of money.

Be receptive to this process and remove money from the situation. Many people have died after leading prosperous but unhappy lives. They now have nothing except anguish to show for it. Money is meaningless. Throw that thinking out the window and follow your genuine passions, and the world will find out how to maintain you. Sustaining, rather than affluent. You will be an exception if your passion occurs to make you rich beyond your wildest expectations. But, if nothing else, you'll be content.

CONCLUSION

I hope this book was able to help you to know how to awaken your Kundalini and Third Eye safely and effectively through meditation. The next step is to keep your chakras burning bright by living a healthy life physically and psychologically.

Remember that Kundalini Awakening is not a one-time affair. It involves keeping yourself fit in body, mind, and spirit. It is natural for energy to revert to its previous levels if you fall back to your old lifestyle and indulge in harmful things. That does not mean that your Kundalini will become dormant once more; it will only manifest itself less strongly than when you have maintained the purity of your energetic channels.

If you have relapsed, review this book and practice its suggestions. When you do, you will experience the full benefits of the Kundalini.

Be with spiritual people – their energies will affect yours. Avoid those with unclean or negative energy if you can. Of course, you may be unable to stay away from them, especially if you live or work with them, but at the very least, protect yourself by imagining a shield around you so their energy fields won't contaminate you.

This book explains the true powers of the Third Eye and the good it may accomplish. It goes into great depth on how to activate the Third Eye. You will learn about pineal gland decalcification and activating our seven chakras. It is widely acknowledged that they have the potential to benefit humanity as a whole. Nonetheless, they remain cloaked in mystery.

This book aims to clarify these concepts and brings you one step closer to understanding them. It places a strong emphasis on the healing abilities of the Third Eye, often known as the Ajna Chakra. It describes the relationship between the Third Eye and the pineal gland and the spiritual consciousness they may provide.

This book will guide you through the process of awakening your Third Eye. It tells you about the wonders that await you along the way. It takes you on this fantastic adventure. The road of meditation leads to the Third Eye's activation.

Most of our sorrows, pain, and suffering are caused by our tension, worry, and uncertainties. They generate negative energies and suffocate our reasoning and consciousness. You've learned how to combat these evils and live a calm and peaceful life – a life with so much to offer and no need to take anything away from anyone. It aids you in achieving inner peace.

Every day, set aside some time to meditate. Concentrate on the Third Eye. Try to rouse it. Recognize its abilities. You may accomplish this using the methods outlined in the book. You can also unleash certain wonderful powers that have always been present in you. It takes you on an incredible adventure — the path to happiness.

Made in the USA
Las Vegas, NV
21 July 2022

51951321R00129